# Neurology

*Editor*

PAULA M. GREGORY

# PRIMARY CARE:
# CLINICS IN OFFICE PRACTICE

www.primarycare.theclinics.com

*Consulting Editor*

JOEL J. HEIDELBAUGH

June 2015 • Volume 42 • Number 2

ELSEVIER

1600 John F. Kennedy Boulevard • Suite 1800 • Philadelphia, Pennsylvania, 19103-2899

http://www.theclinics.com

PRIMARY CARE: CLINICS IN OFFICE PRACTICE Volume 42, Number 2
June 2015 ISSN 0095-4543, ISBN-13: 978-0-323-38904-4

Editor: Jessica McCool
Developmental Editors: Colleen Viola

*Primary Care: Clinics in Office Practice* (ISSN: 0095–4543) is published quarterly by Elsevier Inc., 360 Park Avenue South, New York, NY 10010-1710. Months of issue are March, June, September, and December. Periodicals postage paid at New York, NY and additional mailing offices. Subscription prices are $225.00 per year (US individuals), $392.00 (US institutions), $115.00 (US students), $275.00 (Canadian individuals), $444.00 (Canadian institutions), $175.00 (Canadian students), $345.00 (international individuals), $444.00 (international institutions), and $175.00 (international students). Foreign air speed delivery is included in all *Clinics* subscription prices. All prices are subject to change without notice. POSTMASTER: Send address changes to *Primary Care: Clinics in Office Practice*, Elsevier Periodicals Customer Service, 11830 Westline Industrial Drive, St. Louis, MO 63146. Customer Service Health Sciences Division, Subscription Customer Service, 3251 Riverport Lane, Maryland Heights, MO 63043. **Customer Service: 1-800-654-2452 (U.S. and Canada); 314-447-8871 (outside U.S. and Canada). Fax: 314-447-8029. E-mail: journalscustomerservice-usa@elsevier.com (for print support); journalsonlinesupport-usa@elsevier.com (for online support).**

*Reprints.* For copies of 100 or more, of articles in this publication, please contact the Commercial Reprints Department, Elsevier Inc., 360 Park Avenue South, New York, NY 10010-1710. Tel. 212-633-3874; Fax: 212-633-3820; E-mail: reprints@elsevier.com.

*Primary Care: Clinics in Office Practice* is covered in *MEDLINE/PubMed (Index Medicus)* and *EMBASE/Excerpta Medica, Current Contents/Clinical Medicine,* and *ISI/BIOMED.*

# Contributors

## CONSULTING EDITOR

**JOEL J. HEIDELBAUGH, MD, FAAFP, FACG**
Clinical Associate Professor, Departments of Family Medicine and Urology; Clerkship Director, University of Michigan Medical School, Ann Arbor; Ypsilanti Health Center, Ypsilanti, Michigan

## EDITOR

**PAULA M. GREGORY, DO, MBA**
Assistant Dean of Clinical Education, Georgia Campus of the Philadelphia College of Osteopathic Medicine, Suwannee, Georgia

## AUTHORS

**VIBHUTI ANSAR, MD**
Program Director, Transitional Year Residency; Associate Director, Family Medicine Residency; Columbus Regional Healthcare, Columbus, Georgia

**CHERYL BASDEN, DO, MBA**
Part-time Assistant Professor, Clinical Education, Georgia Campus of the Philadelphia College of Osteopathic Medicine, Suwanee, Georgia

**KIMBERLY BATES, MD, FACP, FAAP**
Program Director, Internal Medicine Residency, Gwinnett Medical Center, Lawrenceville, Georgia

**ROBERT DANOFF, DO, MS, FACOFP, FAAFP**
Program Director, Family Medicine Residency; Program Director, Combined Family Medicine/Emergency Medicine Residency, Aria Health System, Philadelphia, Pennsylvania

**MARK D. DARROW, MD, FACP**
Clinical Professor of General Internal Medicine, Georgia Campus of the Philadelphia College of Osteopathic Medicine, Gwinnett Health Systems, Lawrenceville, Georgia

**DANIEL KANE FILES, DO**
Resident, Family Medicine Residency, Aria Health, Philadelphia, Pennsylvania

**TOMIA PALMER HARMON, MD**
Director of Primary Care Skills, Department of Clinical Education, Georgia Campus of the Philadelphia College of Osteopathic Medicine, Suwanee, Georgia

**JAMES D. HOGUE, DO, FAAEM**
Clinical Assistant Professor of Emergency Medicine, Georgia Campus of the Philadelphia College of Osteopathic Medicine, Suwanee, Georgia

**TANI JAUSURAWONG, DO**
Resident, Combined Internal Medicine/Emergency Medicine Residency, Aria Health,
Philadelphia, Pennsylvania

**KEVIN E. JOHNSON, MD, FAAFP**
Program Director, Family Medicine Residency, Gwinnett Medical Center, Lawrenceville,
Georgia

**RUBA KATRAJIAN, DO**
Resident, Family Medicine Residency, Aria Health, Philadelphia, Pennsylvania

**SHAWN PHILLIPS, MD**
Lancaster General Hospital Family and Community Medicine, Lancaster, Pennsylvania

**NOJAN VALADI, MD**
St. Francis Neurology, Columbus, Georgia

**DEREK WOESSNER, MD, FAAFP**
Associate Director, Lancaster General Hospital Family and Community Medicine,
Lancaster, Pennsylvania

# Contents

Daniel Kane Files, Tani Jausurawong, Ruba Katrajian, and Robert Danoff

> Multiple sclerosis (MS) is a chronic, debilitating disease that can have devastating effects. Presentation varies widely in symptoms, pace, and progression. In addition to a thorough history and physical examination, diagnostic tools required to diagnose MS and exclude other diagnoses include MRI, evoked potential testing, and cerebrospinal fluid analysis. Although the disease is not curable presently, quality of life can be improved by minimizing the frequency and severity of disease burden. Disease modification, symptom management, preservation of function, and treatment of psychosocial issues are paramount to enhance the quality of life for the patient affected with MS.

Nojan Valadi

> Motor neuron diseases can cause progressive impairment of voluntary muscles of movement, respiration, speech, and swallowing. This review discusses the most common motor neuron disease, amyotrophic lateral sclerosis (ALS). It reviews the evaluation, diagnosis, and management of ALS, and its epidemiology, pathophysiology, and management. A coordinated approach by the primary care physician and neurologist is necessary with a focus on treatment options, durable medical equipment needs, and end-of-life discussions.

Vibhuti Ansar and Nojan Valadi

> Guillain-Barré syndrome and its clinical variants are a group of rapidly progressing, potentially debilitating neurologic disorders that may have significant morbidity/mortality if left unrecognized or untreated. The most common symptoms include ascending limb weakness and paralysis, which may progress to respiratory failure. Diagnosis is made clinically with laboratory testing. Several treatment options exist, including plasma exchange and intravenous immunoglobulin administration. Most cases may resolve without sequelae, but those that do not may leave behind significant persistent debility.

Mark D. Darrow

As the population ages, fear of memory loss and potential diagnosis of dementia increases. Primary care providers, with their medical knowledge, familiarity with patients and their loved ones, and knowledge of the community and its resources, are perfectly placed to diagnose and treat commonly presenting types of dementia. As knowledge of the types of dementia and their categorization, presentation, and course has increased, diagnosis and treatment of this problem have become more understandable and amenable to primary care intervention. Diagnosis and work-up use common techniques and studies to assist providers. Treatment and management have evolved over time to include nonpharmacologic or behavioral interventions.

Kevin E. Johnson

Parkinson disease (PD) is a progressive neurodegenerative disease with motor, nonmotor, and behavioral findings. Imaging technology advances have allowed the characterization of the underlying pathologic changes to the brain and identification of specific lesions in dopaminergic neurons. Although certain imaging techniques allow for detection up to 20 years before the onset of motor symptoms, these advances have yet to produce meaningful treatments to halt the disease or reverse its course. Current treatments are directed at optimizing symptomatic management. Referral to a movement disorder specialist familiar with PD should be considered for providers with limited familiarity in diagnosis or treatment.

Kimberly Bates

Although epilepsy has a prevalence of 5 to 7 per 1000 persons in the United States, it continues to be a poorly understood condition. Given the number of patients in the United States with epilepsy, it is very likely that primary care physicians will continue to provide care for these patients. This article refreshes some of the knowledge around the diagnosis of epilepsy, discusses special populations that may require additional management considerations, highlights the association of epilepsy with multiple comorbidities, and discusses antiepileptic drug (AED) treatment, including issues surrounding adherence and safety of AED therapy.

Tomia Palmer Harmon

Migraine headache is a neurologic disorder that occurs in 18% of women and 6% of men. Adults and children with mild to moderate migraine headaches seeking acute therapy should be treated with nonsteroidal anti-inflammatory drugs because of the efficacy, cost, and decreased side effects. Some children and adults require preventive therapy (those with headaches lasting >12 h, those patients with >4 headaches in 1 month, those with headaches that affect their ability to function). Studies have shown that early treatment with large doses of medication work well for the treatment of moderate to severe migraine headache.

Concussions have garnered more attention in the medical literature, media, and social media. As such, in the nomenclature according to the Centers for Disease Control and Prevention, the term *concussion* has been supplanted by the term *mild traumatic brain injury*. Current numbers indicate that 1.7 million TBIs are documented annually, with estimates around 3 million annually (173,285 sports- and recreation-related TBIs among children and adolescents). The Sideline Concussion Assessment Tool 3 and the NFL Sideline Concussion Assessment Tool are commonly used sideline tools.

Patients presenting to primary care with complaints of dizziness are common. Differentiating the cause of dizziness can be made easier by considering 4 main categories of dizziness: vertigo, presyncope/syncope, disequilibrium, and nonspecific symptoms. Differentials should immediately include the most common causes of dizziness, such as benign paroxysmal positional vertigo and orthostatic hypotension. Diagnostic tests should be ordered for patients who have abnormal findings on physical examination that may indicate a more serious cause of dizziness.

Patients who present with mixed clinical neurologic signs and symptoms can be sorted into groups based on the symptom format. Targeted physical examination and evaluation of laboratory results can help quickly segment patients into groups for further workup or admission. The possibility of medication- or toxin-induced neurologic causes must be considered. Medication- and toxin-induced neurologic syndrome is a combination of several symptoms that are induced either by the exposure to or withdrawal of various medications or by toxins, and the symptoms are sometimes difficult to fit into a nice, neat diagnostic package.

# PRIMARY CARE:
# CLINICS IN OFFICE PRACTICE

---

**RELATED INTEREST**

*Neurologic Clinics*, February 2015 (Vol. 33, Issue 1)
**Movement Disorders**
Joseph Jankovic, *Editor*
Available at: http://www.neurologic.theclinics.com/

---

**THE CLINICS ARE AVAILABLE ONLINE!**
Access your subscription at:
www.theclinics.com

# Foreword

# Neurologic Puzzles

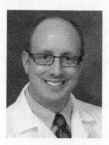

Joel J. Heidelbaugh, MD, FAAFP, FACG
*Consulting Editor*

To many clinicians, there is probably no organ system in the human body more complicated and more intimidating than the nervous system. While medical diagnostics and therapeutics continue to advance, the ability to quickly and accurately diagnose, moreover to prevent or cure, many neurologic conditions remains somewhat elusive. The detailed neurologic examination requires substantial skill and practice over years of experience coupled with a keen insight of when to consider metabolic and radiographic workups and specialty referrals. Also, raising "the proverbial bar" on complexity, many neurologic conditions commonly overlap with psychiatric, endocrine, cardiovascular, metabolic, and genetic disorders.

I recently saw a 72-year-old man in my practice who has been my patient for well over a decade. He presented alone, and I immediately noticed that something was different from my previous interactions with him, but I couldn't exactly pinpoint what was different. He stated that recently he had been more confused, was forgetting where he left his keys and personal items, and had recently fallen twice because he "tripped over his feet." Then, he told me that his wife had been complaining that she could no longer read his handwriting and he was forgetting their friends' names. His medical history is significant for having type 2 diabetes mellitus for over 30 years, hypertension, hyperlipidemia, metabolic syndrome, and an accidental closed head injury in his late 50s that led to early retirement. Both of his parents died from "old age," which he defined as "you know, there were just demented, and sputtered around the nursing home." Prior to his appointment, he took the liberty of researching his symptoms on the Internet and was concerned that he may have had a stroke, or may have amyotrophic lateral sclerosis or early-stage dementia. Then, he handed me a note from his wife, who expressed her concern that he may also have sequelae from his closed head injury or Parkinson disease. While it was unfortunate to see my patient in this state, it certainly presented an interesting diagnostic dilemma on where to start the workup.

Prim Care Clin Office Pract 42 (2015) ix–x
http://dx.doi.org/10.1016/j.pop.2015.03.002
0095-4543/15/$ – see front matter © 2015 Published by Elsevier Inc.

primarycare.theclinics.com

This issue of *Primary Care: Clinics in Office Practice* explores the wide spectrum of neurologic diseases in a comprehensive format of evidence- and guideline-based articles that highlights both acute and chronic conditions. The articles on the chronic conditions of multiple sclerosis, amyotrophic lateral sclerosis, Parkinson disease, and Guillain-Barré syndrome provide an in-depth opportunity to review the diagnosis and therapeutic strategies in managing these conditions. Additional articles detail guideline-based approaches to the management of epilepsy, dementia, dizziness, migraines, and brain injury that outline novel pharmacotherapeutic strategies. A unique article highlighting medication and toxin-induced neurologic symptoms will guide readers toward a critical appraisal of different diagnoses relative to patients in their practices.

The future will see advances in genetic screening and therapies that will allow clinicians to achieve earlier diagnoses for neurologic conditions, and, it is hoped, to offer a novel avenue for therapy in improving quality of life. I offer my gratitude to Dr Paula Gregory and all of the authors who valiantly researched the current literature and wrote informative articles for this issue. I trust that our readers will enjoy this issue as much as I have, and augment their diagnostic and clinical skills in their efforts toward solving "the neurologic puzzles" in their practices.

Joel J. Heidelbaugh, MD, FAAFP, FACG
Departments of Family Medicine and Urology
Department of Family Medicine
University of Michigan Medical School
Ann Arbor, MI 48109, USA

Ypsilanti Health Center
200 Arnet Suite 200
Ypsilanti, MI 48198, USA

E-mail address:
jheidel@umich.edu

# Preface

# Neurologic Diseases: The Tragedy and the Hope

This issue of *Primary Care: Clinics in Office Practice* is dedicated to the neurologic challenges faced by each of us on a daily basis in our practices. You will find represented here issues that require diagnostic and management acumen. Neurologic syndromes may also represent overwhelming situations for the patient, family, and community.

The tragedy of these diseases also saps our emotional energy as we put full efforts in our care of the patients. Our patients challenge and test our ability to maintain and improve the lives of all as they travel through the stages of these illnesses. The responsibility is ours for care of the patient and to improve the lives of all touched by these diseases. Fortunately, there have been tremendous advances in the recent years that give us hope that we can look to the future for new therapy and diagnosis.

Diagnosis and management of dizziness and related problems involve a myriad of potential life-threatening problems that must be diagnosed quickly. Critical thinking and quick action are needed to not miss a medication or a toxic-induced neurologic syndrome. Reviewing medication and toxin-induced neurologic problems keeps our index of suspicion up with the ever-increasing medications that patients take, including over-the-counter medication. This article gives us a quick way to review the nature of the symptom complex.

Migraines and epilepsy are everyday occurrences in the primary care practice and the hope is that we can find a suitable treatment. New medications have improved the patient's life in returning to daily activity as quickly as possible.

Progressive diseases such as Parkinson's and dementia are no longer only diseases of the aged. We see these increasingly in younger patients; with the rapid research cycles, improvements could reach our practices in short time.

Multiple sclerosis, amyotrophic lateral sclerosis, and Guillain-Barré articles give promise and hope to the diseases and diagnosis that have impacted the lives of the patient, family, and community. Our hope is to quickly assist the family and community in care while instituting the most current medical advice.

It has been a distinct pleasure and honor to review these topics and to find new ways of looking at the diseases presented by this issue of *Primary Care: Clinics in Office Practice*. As with all things, we rely on our peers and friends, old and new, to teach us and to be a resource. I am very grateful to have the support of these fine educators and the series consulting editor, Dr Heidelbaugh, for his support and advice. This issue

Prim Care Clin Office Pract 42 (2015) xi–xii
http://dx.doi.org/10.1016/j.pop.2015.03.001
0095-4543/15/$ – see front matter © 2015 Published by Elsevier Inc.

primarycare.theclinics.com

could not exist if it were not for the tireless work by Ms Viola, Ms McCool, and others at Elsevier. I am deeply appreciative of the skill of these fine professionals.

Paula M. Gregory, DO, MBA
Georgia Campus of the
Philadelphia College of Osteopathic Medicine
625 Old Peachtree Road
Suwannee, GA 30026, USA

E-mail address:
Paulagr@pcom.edu

# Multiple Sclerosis

Daniel Kane Files, DO, Tani Jausurawong, DO, Ruba Katrajian, DO,
Robert Danoff, DO, MS*

## KEYWORDS

- Multiple sclerosis • Vitamin D • Epstein–Barr virus • Latitude

## KEY POINTS

- Multiple sclerosis is a chronic and debilitating disease that can have many devastating effects physically and psychologically.
- Although certain clinical features are typical of MS, the presentation of the disease varies widely in symptoms as well as in pace and progression.
- In addition to a thorough history and physical examination, diagnostic tools required to diagnose MS and exclude other diagnoses include MRI, evoked potential testing, and cerebrospinal fluid analysis.
- Although MS is not curable at this point, quality of life can be improved by minimizing the frequency and severity of disease burden.
- Disease modification, symptom management, preservation of function, and treatment of psychosocial issues are paramount to enhance the quality of life for the patient.

## INTRODUCTION
### Disease Description

Multiple sclerosis (MS) is a chronic disease characterized by multifocal inflammation, demyelination, gliosis, and neuronal loss of the brain and spinal cord. MS affects approximately 400,000 individuals in the United States and affects 2.5 million individuals worldwide,[1] varying greatly with geography. The incidence peaks at 30 years old and the prevalence peaks at 50.[2] Patients present with neurologic findings disseminated in space and time, that is affecting differing locations and occurring over multiple episodes. The manifestations of the disease vary greatly, ranging from benign findings to rapidly evolving with the potential for incapacitating disease progression. The course of the disease may be relapsing–remitting, primary progressive, or secondary progressive. The latter is progression after an initial relapsing–remitting phase. Life expectancy in the MS population is reduced by 7 to 14 years compared with the general, healthy population.[3]

Family Medicine Residency, Combined Family Medicine/Emergency Medicine Residency, Aria Health, Red Lion and Knights Roads, Philadelphia, PA 19114, USA
* Corresponding author.
E-mail address: rdanoff@ariahealth.org

Prim Care Clin Office Pract 42 (2015) 159–175
http://dx.doi.org/10.1016/j.pop.2015.01.007
0095-4543/15/$ – see front matter © 2015 Elsevier Inc. All rights reserved.

## Summary/Discussion

MS occurrence varies greatly across the world. It is predominantly found throughout Europe, southern Canada, northern US, New Zealand and southeastern Australia (**Fig. 1**). For many of these areas, the prevalence is around 100 per 100,000, which is that of the United States.[4] The greatest prevalence reported is 300 per 100,000 in the Orkney Islands, off northern Scotland.[4] There is limited incidence of the disease in Africa, Mexico, Puerto Rico, Japan, China, and Philippines, as well as in the Native American population.[5] Because of the focused distribution, many studies have focused on the risk factors in an attempt to determine a potential link as to the cause(s) of the disease.

Genetic susceptibility to the disease is readily apparent with the 15 to 35 times greater risk in first-degree relatives of those with the disease.[5] Although the general population has a prevalence rate of 1 per 1000, monozygotic twins have a rate of 270 per 1000 (**Table 1**).[6] Interestingly a study completed on half-siblings found that the risk for maternal half-siblings was 2.35% compared with 1.31% for paternal half-siblings, alluding to a substantial maternal effect in transmission.[5] The strongest genetic effect in MS seems to be the major human histocompatibility system, a region on chromosome 6, responsible for the HLA-DRB1 allele.[5,7] This area plays a role in creating human leukocyte antigens that present to T cells and may trigger an immune response. The interaction is complex and it is still unclear as to the exact role that interaction may play in the disease process. However, it is known to be associated with other autoimmune diseases, namely, rheumatoid arthritis, type 1 diabetes, sarcoid, and pemphigus.[8]

Although genetics are known to be linked to the development of MS, that does not explain or account for all cases of this disease. Additional risk factors have been identified as having a direct or causal link to MS, including latitude, vitamin D level, and Epstein–Barr virus (**Table 2**).

Latitude: In areas of temperate climate, there is an increase in the incidence of MS the further north from the equator with increasing latitude.[9] Interestingly, studies of immigrant populations found that those who migrated before adolescence acquired

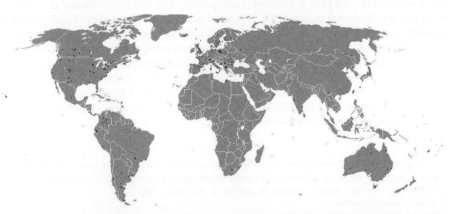

**Fig. 1.** World map showing the distribution of all prevalence estimates included in this meta-analysis. (*From* Simpson S Jr, Blizzard L, Otahal P, et al. Latitude is significantly associated with the prevalence of multiple sclerosis: a meta-analysis. J Neurol Neurosurg Psychiatry 2011;82(10):1136; with permission.)

**Table 1**
**Population-based prevalence rates in relatives of MS probands**

| Population | Prevalence |
|---|---|
| General population rate | 1/1000 |
| Adoptive siblings | 1/1000 |
| First cousin | 7/1000 |
| Paternal half sibling | 13/1000 |
| Half sibling reared apart | 21/1000 |
| Maternal half sibling | 24/1000 |
| Full sibling risk | 35/1000 |
| HLA identical sibling | 80/1000 |
| Sibling in consanguineous mating | 90/1000 |
| Child or sibling | 197/1000 |
| Offspring conjugal pair | 200/1000 |
| Monozygotic twin risk | 270/1000 |

*From* Ebers GC. Environmental factors and multiple sclerosis. Lancet Neurol 2008;7(3):272; with permission.

the risk of their new country, whereas those who migrated after adolescence retained the risk of their home country location.[5]

Vitamin D level: The geographic variability and distance from the equator has raised questions as to the relationship between sunlight and vitamin D levels in the disease process. Levels of estimated sun exposure time during childhood and adolescence are inversely related to MS susceptibility. When looking at areas in high latitudes, populations with diets high in vitamin D–rich, fatty fish had lower than expected prevalence for the latitude in which they reside.[7] Even more evidence for vitamin D involvement came from a prospective nested case-control study in United States–based military personnel associating a lower risk of disease with high serum 25-hydroxyvitamin D levels. Additionally, it was found that participants had lower serum vitamin D levels during MS flares than when they were in remission, and that the level of deficiency correlated with the disease severity (**Fig. 2**).[7]

Season of birth: In Canada, the UK, Sweden, and Denmark, the highest rates of MS occurred in people born in of May and the lowest occurred in those born during

**Table 2**
**Risk factors for multiple sclerosis**

| Environmental | Genetic |
|---|---|
| Europe, Russia, southern Canada, northern US, New Zealand, Southeast Australia | HLA-DRB1 on chromosome 6 |
| Latitude >40° north | First-degree relative |
| Migration before adolescence to high-risk area, or migration after adolescence from a high-risk area<br>Birth in May<br>Low vitamin D levels<br>Smoking<br>Epstein–Barr virus (more so in adolescents and adults)<br>Obesity | Maternal > paternal effect |

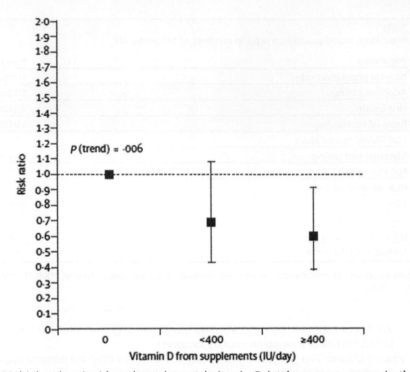

**Fig. 2.** Multiple sclerosis risk and supplemental vitamin D intake among women in the Nurses Health Studies. (*From* Ascherio A, Munger KL. Environmental risk factors for multiple sclerosis. part II: noninfectious factors. Ann Neurol 2007;61(6):505; with permission.)

November.[5,7] A potential theory is that the low level of sunlight exposure during the winter months of a pregnancy before a May birth lead to low vitamin D levels and put the child at increased risk, whereas the summer months leading up to a November birth provided increased vitamin D and offered a protective effect to the unborn child. Although a protective level of vitamin D intake has not yet been established, it was noted with supplementation of as little as 400 IU or greater the incidence of the development of MS was 41% lower compared with those without vitamin D supplementation.[7]

Epstein–Barr virus: There is a potential correlation of previous infection with Epstein–Barr virus and the development of MS. Those with higher titers of anti–Epstein–Barr virus antibodies may have increased risk than those with lower titers, but the significance of this finding is unknown.[5] However, those who are infected with Epstein–Barr virus at an older age tend to have more severe symptoms, and some studies have linked the age of infectivity with an increased risk for the development of MS.[10] This may be owing to the number of CD8$^+$ T cells one has when first exposed to the Epstein–Barr virus; children have higher levels and are less likely to have progression to mononucleosis, whereas adolescents and adults have lower levels making infectivity more severe and allowing for an autoimmune cascade to ensue.[10]

Smoking: A dose-dependent relationship has been observed in smokers, with an increasing number of cigarettes correlating with a higher risk for MS.[5,11] In fact, multiple studies on US women smokers have shown a 60% greater incidence of MS compared with those women that have never smoked.[11]

## MULTIPLE SCLEROSIS DIAGNOSIS

MS is a chronic, degenerative disease of the central nervous system that is thought to be autoimmune in nature. Its inflammatory process attacks the brain and spinal cord, and is the most common neurologically disabling disease in young adults. Although genetics contribute to its cause, environmental factors are also thought to play an important role in triggering the disease process.

## PATHOLOGY

MS is a demyelinating disease of the central nervous system whose cause continues to elude us. However, the current theory proposes that the disease begins with an inflammatory autoimmune process that results in the formation of the histopathologic hallmark — plaques.[12-14] Additionally, it seems that a combination of genetic predisposition and environmental insult is needed to trigger development of the disease. Studies have shown that there is a mildly increased concordance rate of MS among monozygotic twins of 20% to 35%, suggesting that environmental effects play a large role.[6]

The plaque of MS is thought to result from a breach in the blood–brain barrier caused by upregulation of adhesion molecules on the endothelium of the brain and spinal cord, which allows leukocytes to traverse the vessel walls. Once T cells enter the central nervous system, they react with myelin antigens and cause an inflammatory demyelination. This reaction leads to increased macrophage and microglial activity that results in a loss of the oligodendrocyte/myelin complex and causes axonal damage. With the vulnerability in the blood–brain barrier, B cells also enter the central nervous system. They release both immunoglobulin (Ig)M and IgG antibodies, resulting in the oligoclonal bands that can be detected on agarose gel electrophoresis along with an increased IgG index. It is unknown to what central nervous system antigen these antibodies are being produced.[12] The heterogeneous nature of the disease is also evident in the unpredictable pattern of lesions, as well as in the variability in stage and histology.

Acute, active plaques are prevalent in acute and relapsing–remitting stages, and are abundant in macrophages that contain myelin fragments. Inactive plaques are filled with empty macrophages. Chronic plaques are seen in progressive MS and are characterized by macrophages at the edges with central sparing. They are also completely demyelinated. Despite the cellular differences, some form of inflammation is present in all lesion types; however, with advancing patient age and greater disease duration, the severity of the inflammatory response decreases. It is this inflammation that drives the demyelination and neurodegeneration of the disease process.[14]

## TYPES OF MULTIPLE SCLEROSIS

Relapsing–remitting is the most common diagnostic type of MS. It is more common in women and is characterized by relapses or exacerbations of previous symptoms or the appearance of new ones. After the relapse, a period of full or partial recovery lasts for days, weeks, or months.

Secondary progressive MS is a sequelae of prolonged relapsing/remitting MS. It is characterized by a gradual worsening of the symptoms between relapses. Although there may be short intervals of symptom remission, these periods decrease over time and are often accompanied by a progression of the severity of symptoms.

Progressive relapsing MS tends to increase in severity from the initial disease onset. Although there are periods of remission, each relapse that follows is often characterized by more severe symptoms.

Primary progressive MS is characterized by a gradual progression of the disease without periods of remission. Men and women seem to be equally affected, with the most common age of onset between late 30s and early 40s. Disease activity is more prevalent in the spinal cord and is less likely than other forms to affect cognitive function. Symptom acuity has the potential to level off.

## SYMPTOM SEQUELAE

The diagnosis of MS may be made on clinical grounds alone or by imaging in addition to clinical findings. Symptoms must last for longer than 24 hours per event and occur as distinct episodes that are separated by 1 month or more.[15]

Patients may present with symptoms that are secondary to 1 monofocal solitary central nervous system lesion or have symptoms that are secondary from multifocal lesions located in 2 or more separate regions of the central nervous system. These symptoms may be monophasic with a single occurrence, multiphasic with a relapsing nature, or progressive.

Patients may complain of blurred or double vision, color desaturation or dimness, periorbital pain with eye movement, visual blurring during a hot shower or with physical exertion, weakness of the limbs, exercise-induced weakness, or generalized fatigue. Sensory symptoms in MS vary widely from paresthesias including tingling or prickling sensations, "pins and needles" or painful burning to hypesthesia manifested as reduced sensation, numbness, or even a "dead" feeling. Bladder dysfunction occurs in more than 90% of patients with MS and results in episodes of incontinence in up to one-third of patients, causing social debilitation.[15] Symptoms may also be mild including frequency, urgency, and hesitancy. However, bladder dysfunction secondary to detrusor sphincter dyssynergia results in recurrent urinary tract infections. Cognitive dysfunction is common, usually with impaired attention, difficulty shifting between tasks, and slowed information processing. However, dementia is an uncommon finding.

## DISABILITY STATUS

Several rating scales exist to assist in the measurement of disability from MS. The Expanded Disability Status Score (EDSS) and Functional Systems Scores (FSS) are the most widely used measures of neurologic impairment in MS. The FSS quantifies disability in 7 defined functional systems as well as an additional category for other findings with information obtained by standard neurologic examination. These data are then used in conjunction with observations and information regarding gait and the use of assistive devices to rate the EDSS. The EDSS rating scale ranges in half-point increments from 0 (normal neurologic examination) to 10 (death owing to MS).[16,17] These rating scales are commonly used in clinical trial. However they have less utility in the monitoring of progression of disease especially once patients have ambulatory difficulties.[18]

## DIAGNOSING THE DISEASE

The original diagnostic criteria for MS were previously based on clinical features of demyelination alone.[19] Over time, several criteria have been developed and replaced. As radiologic imaging techniques have advanced, the McDonald criteria have sought to integrate clinical, laboratory and radiographic data in the establishment of MS (Table 3).

## CLINICAL FINDINGS
### Physical Examination

- Hyperreflexia, extensor plantar responses, lower extremity ataxia, impaired rapid alternating movements, loss of vibration, and proprioception
- Cerebellar tremors of the head or trunk, and; cerebellar dysarthria manifested as scanning speech
- Visual loss or afferent pupillary defect secondary to optic neuropathy
- Internuclear ophthalmoplegia, papillitis, and pendular nystagmus
- Intention tremor, spasticity, dysarthria, and paraparesis
- Lhermitte sign
- Ascending paresthesias, bandlike tightness around the torso, and impaired sphincter function secondary to acute myelitis.

### Diagnostic Modalities

MRI is used routinely for decisions regarding treatment, for the detection of subclinical disease, and for prognostication of the course of MS in an individual. Conventional MRI techniques are used currently to diagnose and follow patients with MS. With technological advances, nonconventional MRI techniques are now able to detect changes not seen on conventional MRI and even predict disability (**Table 4**).

### Imaging

Traditionally visualized MS lesions (plaques) fall into the categories of hyperintensities on T2-weighted images and hypointensities on T1-weighted images, and gadolinium-positive lesions.[20] Hyperintensity on T2-weighted MRI indicates alterations in water content and is thus not specific to the underlying pathology. However, lesion location and morphology are helpful in differentiating true demyelinating lesions from lesions of other etiology. For example, MS lesions are usually oval or ovoid in morphology, measuring 5 mm or greater in diameter and are located supratentorially. One-half of acute hypointense lesions on T1-weighted MRI scan revert to an area of T2 signal abnormality, likely representing reversible edema and inflammation. However, the remaining one-half of lesions that last longer than 6 months likely represent irreversible changes, as found in significant demyelination and axonal loss, correlating better than hyperintense T2 lesions with clinical disability. Gadolinium-positive lesions represent T-cell migration across the blood–brain barrier, reflected by intravenous gadolinium leaking into the parenchyma. Gadolinium-positive lesions are more commonly seen in relapsing–remitting MS. Although the morphology of gadolinium-positive lesions can vary greatly, the most indicative lesions of MS are in an incomplete or open ring pattern.[20]

## DIAGNOSTIC DILEMMAS

Many conditions can mimic MS clinically or radiologically. The diagnosis of MS is more difficult early in the disease, when symptoms distributed in time and space are absent and when the disease runs a progressive course without periodic exacerbations. Additionally, MS, systemic lupus erythematosus, and antiphospholipid syndrome are all chronic, immune-mediated disorders with a relapsing–remitting presentation affecting young adults, making differentiation even more problematic. Some red flags that likely point toward a diagnosis other than MS include bone lesions, lung or renal involvement, multiple cranial neuropathies or polyradiculopathy, retinopathy, hematologic manifestations, persistent gadolinium enhancement, and enlargement of lesions.[19,23]

**Table 3**
2010 McDonald criteria for the diagnosis of MS

| Clinical Presentation | Additional Data Needed for MS Diagnosis |
|---|---|
| ≥2 attacks[a], objective clinical evidence of ≥2 lesions or objective clinical evidence of 1 lesion with reasonable historical evidence of a prior attack[b] | None[c] |
| ≥2 attacks[a], objective clinical evidence of 1 lesion | Dissemination in space, demonstrated by ≥1 T2 lesion in ≥2 of 4 MS-typical regions of the CNS (periventricular, juxtacortical, infratentorial, or spinal cord)[d]; or await a further clinical attack[a] implicating a different CNS site |
| 1 attack[a], objective clinical evidence of ≥2 lesions | Dissemination in time, demonstrated by: Simultaneous presence of asymptomatic gadolinium-enhancing and nonenhancing lesions at any time; or a new T2 and/or gadolinium-enhancing lesion(s) on follow-up MRI, irrespective of its timing with reference to a baseline scan; or await a second clinical attack[a] |
| 1 attack[a], objective clinical evidence of 1 lesion (clinically isolated syndrome) | Dissemination in space and time, demonstrated by: For DIS: ≥1 T2 lesion in ≥2 of 4 MS-typical regions of the CNS (periventricular, juxtacortical, infratentorial, or spinal cord)[d]; or Await a second clinical attack[a] implicating a different CNS site; and For DIT: Simultaneous presence of asymptomatic gadolinium-enhancing and nonenhancing lesions at any time; or a new T2 and/or gadolinium-enhancing lesion(s) on follow-up MRI, irrespective of its timing with reference to a baseline scan; or await a second clinical attack[a] |

| Insidious neurological progression suggestive of MS (PPMS) | 1 year of disease progression (retrospectively or prospectively determined) plus 2 of 3 of the following criteria[d]: |
|---|---|
| | 1. Evidence for DIS in the brain based on ≥1 T2 lesions in the MS-characteristic (periventricular, juxtacortical, or infratentorial) regions |
| | 2. Evidence for DIS in the spinal cord based on ≥2 T2 lesions in the cord |
| | 3. Positive CSF (isoelectric focusing evidence of oligoclonal bands and/or elevated IgG index) |

If the criteria are fulfilled and there is no better explanation for the clinical presentation, the diagnosis is "MS"; if suspicious, but the criteria are not completely met, the diagnosis is "possible MS"; if another diagnosis arises during the evaluation that better explains the clinical presentation, then the diagnosis is "not MS." *Abbreviations:* CNS, central nervous system; CSF, cerebrospinal fluid; DIS, dissemination in space; DIT, dissemination in time; IgG, immunoglobulin G; MS, multiple sclerosis; PPMS, primary progressive multiple sclerosis.

[a] An attack (relapse; exacerbation) is defined as patient-reported or objectively observed events typical of an acute inflammatory demyelinating event in the CNS, current or historical, with duration of ≥24 hours, in the absence of fever or infection. It should be documented by contemporaneous neurologic examination, but some historical events with symptoms and evolution characteristic for MS, but for which no objective neurologic findings are documented, can provide reasonable evidence of a prior demyelinating event. Reports of paroxysmal symptoms (historical or current) should, however, consist of multiple episodes occurring over not <24 hours. Before a definite diagnosis of MS can be made, ≥1 attack must be corroborated by findings on neurologic examination, visual evoked potential response in patients reporting prior visual disturbance, or MRI consistent with demyelination in the area of the CNS implicated in the historical report of neurologic symptoms.

[b] Clinical diagnosis based on objective clinical findings for 2 attacks is most secure. Reasonable historical evidence for 1 past attack, in the absence of documented objective neurologic findings, can include historical events with symptoms and evolution characteristics for a prior inflammatory demyelinating event; ≥1 attack, however, must be supported by objective findings.

[c] No additional tests are required. However, it is desirable that any diagnosis of MS be made with access to imaging based on these criteria. If imaging or other tests (eg, CSF) are undertaken and are negative, extreme caution needs to be taken before making a diagnosis of MS, and alternative diagnoses must be considered. There must be no better explanation for the clinical presentation, and objective evidence must be present to support a diagnosis of MS.

[d] Gadolinium-enhancing lesions are not required; symptomatic lesions are excluded from consideration in subjects with brainstem or spinal cord syndromes.

*From* Polman CH, Reingold SC, Banwell B, et al. Diagnostic criteria for multiple sclerosis: 2010 revisions to the McDonald criteria. Ann Neurol 2011;69(2):297; with permission.

**Table 4**
Considerations for diagnostic modalities

| Diagnostic Modality | Considerations |
| --- | --- |
| MRI | The routine evaluation for suspected MS includes the following: conventional spin-echo, noncontrast, axial T1-weighted; T2-weighted; axial and sagittal FLAIR; and postcontrast (Gd1) T1-weighted techniques.[20] |
| VEP testing | EP testing evaluates function of afferent and efferent CNS pathways through the use of computer averaged measurement of CNS electrical potentials that have been evoked by repetitive stimulation of selected peripheral nerves or of the brain. EP abnormalities are not specific to patients with MS, but a marked delay in the latency of a specific EP component indicates demyelination. Eighty percent to 90% of patients with MS may display abnormalities on ≥1 modalities of EP.[15] Abnormal VEPs expected to be seen in MS include delay with a well-preserved waveform. |
| | Visual complaints are common in patients with MS. The frequency of patients with MS will be found to have abnormal VEPs ranging between 42% and 100%,[21] some of which may have no visual complaints. The optic chiasm is affected frequently and a healed lesion results in slowed nerve conduction. For these reasons, it is common for patients to have VEP or visual evoked response testing performed. This test involves having the patient look at a checkerboard pattern that alternates black and white squares. The time between the pattern changing and the time of EEG change over the occipital lobe is measured. If significant discrepancy in time exists between the 2 eyes, an intrinsic problem of the eye, the retina or the optic nerve must be further investigated. SSEPs and BAEPs may also be used for evidence of demyelination. |
| CSF analysis | CSF abnormalities found in MS include mononuclear cell pleocytosis and oligoclonal bands. A mild pleocytosis (slightly elevated protein concentration) of >5 cells/μL is present in approximately 25% of patients, particularly after an acute relapse. A pleocytosis of >75 cells/μL, the presence of polymorphonuclear lymphocytes, or a protein concentration >1 g/L should raise the concern of the patient not having MS. The measurement of oligoclonal bands assesses the synthesis of intrathecal IgG, detected on agarose gel electrophoresis. Elevated IgG and oligoclonal bands are not specific to MS and have been found in a variety of inflammatory disorders.[15,22] |
| | Positive CSF findings of increased IgG index or ≥2 oligoclonal bands were previously used to reduce MRI requirement for establishment of dissemination in space. However, the International Panel on Diagnosis of MS deemed this no longer appropriate in 2010.[19] These CSF findings support the underlying inflammatory demyelinating nature of the disease and can be used to evaluate alternative diagnoses. Further studies are required to confirm the additional diagnostic value of CSF. |

Abbreviations: BAEP, brain stem auditory evoked potential; CNS, central nervous system; EP, evoked potential; FLAIR, fluid-attenuated inversion recovery; Gd1, gadolinium 1; IgG, immunoglobulin G; MS, multiple sclerosis; SSEP, short-latency somatosensory evoked potential; VEP, visual evoked potential.
Data from Refs.[15,19–22]

## Process of Elimination

See **Table 5** for a differential diagnosis of MS.

## Comorbidities

### Psychiatric comorbidities

The lifetime prevalence of depression in patients with MS is 50%,[24] which is 3 times greater than the general population. Additionally, up to 15% of patients attending MS clinics have deaths attributed to suicide.[24] Although the pathophysiology of depression in those with MS is understood poorly, some studies suggest that depressed patients have more lesions at particular regions of the brain. This pattern suggests that depression may be a secondary manifestation of MS,[24] not just a comorbidity. Anxiety, bipolar disorder, and psychosis also have higher rates of occurrence among patients with MS than those in the general population. This correlation is particularly important to clinicians, because corticosteroid administration may transiently cause depression, mania, or psychosis.

### Physical comorbidities

Particular interest has been raised among autoimmune diseases. Some studies have suggested an increased likelihood of specific autoimmune diseases in patients with MS.[24] Although some factors are common between MS and certain autoimmune diseases, other factors may actually be protective against particular autoimmune diseases.[25,26] The most commonly cited comorbidities among patients with MS include irritable bowel syndrome, chronic lung disease, hypertension, hyperlipidemia, and arthritis. Additionally, 40% of patients with MS suffer from insomnia in comparison with 10% to 15% of the general population.[24] This last symptom may be influenced by pain, nocturia, spasticity, mood disturbance, or medication prescribed to treat other symptoms of MS.

The risk of fracture is greater among patients with MS secondary to additional factors that increase their risk of osteoporosis and falls.[24] Although corticosteroid use, immobilization, vitamin D insufficiency, and female sex are risk factors that would predispose those with MS to osteoporosis, there have also been reports of higher than expected rates of osteoporosis among newly diagnosed patients with MS. This correlation between osteoporosis and MS is not completely understood and needs further investigation.

### Substance abuse

Patients with MS often display harmful health behaviors, such as tobacco and alcohol abuse. In fact, nearly 13.6% of MS patients reported concomitant alcohol abuse[24] and 50% of patients reported tobacco smoking before MS symptom onset,[24] although no particular time frame was indicated in this study. Smoking also predisposes this population to other conditions such as osteoporosis, cancer, stroke, and lung disease.

### Inactivity

It has been noted that those with MS are less physically active than the general population, leading to increased obesity and thus several other comorbid conditions. Interestingly, obesity at 20 years of age has been associated with a 2-fold increased risk of MS.[24]

## MULTIPLE SCLEROSIS MANAGEMENT STRATEGIES

Treatment of MS is difficult, because the disease process itself is very complex. Much has changed in the management over the last 20 years, and it will likely continue to

| Table 5 Differential diagnosis of multiple sclerosis | |
|---|---|
| Genetic disorders | Hereditary optic neuritis Hereditary spastic paraparesis Leukodystrophy Mitochondrial diseases Spinocerebellar ataxias Wilson disease |
| Infections | Chronic meningitis HTLV-1 (tropical spastic paraparesis) HIV-associated myelopathy Listeria Lyme disease Neurobrucellosis Neurosyphilis PML Whipple's disease |
| Inflammatory conditions | Behçet disease CNS vasculitis Sarcoidosis Sjögren syndrome Systemic lupus erythematosus Systemic sclerosis Mixed connective tissue disease Myasthenia gravis Neuroretinitis |
| Structural conditions and mass lesions | CNS lymphoma Cervical spondylosis Chiari malformation Herniated disc Platybasia Syringomyelia Spinal cord neoplasms (astrocytoma and ependymomas) Tumors of the foramen magnum and posterior fossa |
| Toxic–metabolic disturbances | Copper deficiency Central pontine myelinolysis Manganese toxicity Nitrous oxide toxicity Vitamin $B_{12}$ deficiency |
| Vascular conditions | Antiphospholipid antibody syndrome CADASIL Cerebrovascular disease Microinfarcts owing to polycythemia vera or thrombocytosis Subacute bacterial endocarditis with recurrent emboli Vascular malformations with recurrent bleeding |
| Other demyelinating diseases | ADEM |

Abbreviations: ADEM, acute disseminated encephalomyelitis; CADASIL, cerebral autosomal dominant arteriopathy with subcortical infarcts and leukoencephalopathy; CNS, central nervous system; HIV, human immunodeficiency virus; HTLV-1, human T-cell lymphotropic virus 1; PML, progressive multifocal leukoencephalopathy.

Data from Refs.[15,19,23]

evolve in the near future. This section highlights the different modalities for the treatment of MS, as well as their associated risks and benefits.

## Management Goals

Because there is no cure presently for MS, the treatment is divided into a 2-pronged approach: disease-modifying medications and symptom management.

## Pharmacologic Strategies

### Disease-modifying medications

1. The interferons were the first approved category of medications for the relapsing forms of MS.[27] Differing in their routes of delivery and duration of action, interferons have a complex mechanism of action that is not entirely understood, but is thought to prevent inflammatory cells from crossing the blood–brain barrier.[27] They have been shown to decrease relapse rate and disease burden on imaging, but they do not slow disease progression.[27] Major side effects include flulike symptoms (can be mitigated with pretreatment and posttreatment nonsteroidal antiinflammatory drugs), as well as depression, local skin reactions, allergic reactions, and liver abnormalities. Released in 1993, interferon beta 1b (Betaseron 0.25 mg SC every other day) was the first medication of this category released and is a daily subcutaneous injection. Interferon beta 1A (Avonex 30 mcg IM weekly) is an intramuscular injection given once per week. The prefilled syringes require refrigeration. The subcutaneous form of interferon beta 1A (Rebif 44 mcg SC 3 times per week) is given 3 times per week, but may cause increased skin irritation.
2. Glatiramer acetate (Copaxone 20 mg SC daily or 40 mg SC 3X/week) is a first-line treatment given daily by subcutaneous injection that is indicated for the relapsing–remitting form of MS. The US Food and Drug Administration also approved recently treatments with higher doses 3 times per week.[28] Studies have shown this be effective in decreasing the number of clinical exacerbations.[27] Its mechanism of action is not completely understood, but is thought to enhance specific antiinflammatory Th2 cytokines.[27] Although copaxone may not have the flulike symptoms associated with the interferons, it is accompanied with local skin reactions as well as a postmedication syndrome involving shortness of breath, chest tightness, and flushing that may last 30 seconds to 30 minutes.
3. Natalizumab (Tysabri 300 mg IV every 4 weeks) is thought to block the transmigration of lymphocytes across the blood–brain barrier[27] and is a monotherapeutic intravenous infusion required every 4 weeks at a registered facility for the treatment of relapsing MS. Although it has been shown to reduce the risk of sustained progression of disability and the rate of clinical relapse,[29] it has been associated with progressive multifocal leukoencephalopathy when the patient has anti-JC virus antibodies, prior use of immunosuppressants, and/or an increased duration of treatment.[30] Therefore, the patient must be monitored for the JC virus before starting therapy and can only be used if a patient has had 1 or more relapses in the past year as well as failure or intolerance to alternative first-line medications.[31] Other common side effects include headache, fatigue, urinary tract infections, and joint and chest pain.
4. Fingolimod (Gilenya 0.5 mg oral daily) is thought to sequester lymphocytes in lymph nodes.[27] It is the first daily oral medication approved for the treatment of relapsing forms of MS in those with a relapse within the past year in addition to evidence that alternative disease-modifying medications have been ineffective or tolerated poorly.[32] Studies have demonstrated that Fingolimod decreases the rate of relapse, the cumulative probability of progression of disability, and lesion burden

on MRI against placebo. It has demonstrated a decreased relapse rate when compared with the interferon class of medications.[32]

5. Teriflunomide (Aubagio 7-14 mg oral daily) is a daily oral agent that reduces B- and T-cell activation, proliferation, and function in response to autoantigens. It has been shown to reduce relapse rates, disability progression, and MRI evidence of disease activity.[33] Side effects include abnormal liver function tests, hair loss, gastrointestinal issues, and immunosuppression.

6. Mitoxantrone (Novantrone 12 mg/m$^2$ IV every 3 months) is an immunosuppressant that decreases neurologic disability. It is administered as a 4 times per year intravenous infusion (maximum of 8–12 doses) and is indicated for the progressive, relapsing–remitting forms of MS. It is currently the only drug approved for the progressive forms of MS. However, its use is limited owing to dose-dependent cardiotoxicity, as well leukopenia, alopecia, and liver function abnormalities.[27]

7. Dimethyl fumarate (Tecfidera 240 mg oral two times daily) is approved as a first-line treatment of relapsing MS. It is a twice daily oral pill that is thought to possess anti-inflammatory and cytoprotective properties.[34] It has been shown to decrease the frequency of relapses and improve neuroradiologic outcomes.[34] Side effects include flushing, proteinuria, decrease in white blood cell counts, liver function abnormalities, and gastrointestinal issues.

## Symptom Management

Acute exacerbations of MS are managed with 3 to 5 days of high-dose corticosteroids, but other options include adrenocorticotrophic hormone or plasmapheresis for those who cannot tolerate steroids or are refractory to treatment.[35] MS can have a wide range of symptoms that can be treated individually. Although physical, speech, and occupational therapy can all be useful in coping with disabilities, medications can be used to treat secondary symptoms such as spasticity, pain, bladder dysfunction, depression, and fatigue as noted in **Table 6**.

## Symptomatic Therapies for Multiple Sclerosis

### Nonpharmacologic strategies

The mainstay of treatment for MS is centered around medication management; however, nonpharmacologic modalities can also be beneficial for symptom management.

| Table 6 Symptomatic treatments | |
|---|---|
| **Symptom** | **Treatments** |
| Spasticity | Muscle relaxants: baclofen, dantrolene, cyclobenzaprine, metaxalone, tizanidine |
| Bladder urgency | Antispasmodics: oxybutynin, tolterodine, solifenacin, hyoscyamine |
| Erectile dysfunction | Vardenafil, sildenafil, tadalafil |
| Pain and paroxysmal disorder | Duloxetine, carbamazepine, amitriptyline, gabapentin, nortriptyline, pregabalin |
| Depression | SSRIs, SNRIs, bupropion, tricyclic antidepressants |
| Fatigue | SSRIs, symmetrel, provigil |

*Abbreviations:* SNRI, serotonin and norepinephrine reuptake inhibitor; SSRI, selective serotonin reuptake inhibitor.

*Data from* Calabresi P. Diagnosis and management of multiple sclerosis. Am Fam Physician 2004;70(10):1935–44.

The goal of these therapies is to maximize functionality and quality of life. For mobility deficits, physical therapy as well as integrative medicine such as acupuncture can be used to treat spasticity or weakness. Osteopathic manipulative therapy can also be used in this regard. Special types of orthotics or other devices to aid with movement can be beneficial.[36] As with any chronic disease, psychological issues may arise. It is important to recognize this secondary complication and treat with medication and/or therapy.

*Prognosis*

There is no current cure and affected patients have a decrease in life expectancy by about 7 to 14 years. There is great variation in the severity of exacerbations as well as the rapidity of the accumulation of disability. Patients may exhibit exacerbations that rapidly expand their disability or may experience symptoms that are more mild in nature. Because treatment response varies from person to person, the ultimate management goal should be tailored to preserve patient functionality and quality of life for as long as possible, including decreasing exacerbations as well as disease burden.

## SUMMARY/DISCUSSION

MS is a chronic and debilitating disease that can have many devastating effects physically and psychologically. Although certain clinical features are typical of MS, presentation varies widely in symptoms as well as in pace and progression. In addition to a thorough history and physical examination, diagnostic tools required to diagnose MS and exclude other diagnoses include MRI, evoked potential testing, and cerebrospinal fluid analysis. Although the disease is not curable presently, quality of life can be improved greatly by attempting to minimize the frequency and severity of disease burden. Disease modification, symptom management, preservation of function, and treatment of psychosocial issues are all paramount to enhance the quality of life for the patient affected with MS.

## REFERENCES

1. MS Overview. What is multiple sclerosis? Multiple Sclerosis Association of America; Web. 01 Mar 2015. Available at: http://mymsaa.org/about-ms/overview/#WhoGetsMS.
2. Koch-Henriksen N, Sorensen PS. The changing demographic pattern of multiple sclerosis epidemiology. Lancet Neurol 2010;9:520–32.
3. Scalfari A, Knappertz V, Cutter G, et al. Mortality in patients with multiple sclerosis. Neurology 2013;81:184–92.
4. Olek MJ. Epidemiology and clinical features of multiple sclerosis in adults. UpTo-Date; 2013. Web. 26 Jan. 2014. Available at: http://www.uptodate.com/contents/pathogenesis-and-epidemiology-of-multiple-sclerosis?source=see_link.
5. Ramagopalan SV, Sadovnick AD. Epidemiology of multiple sclerosis. Neurol Clin 2011;29:207–17.
6. Ebers GC. Environmental factors and multiple sclerosis. Lancet Neurol 2008;7:268–77.
7. Ascherio A, Munger KL, Simon KC. Vitamin D and multiple sclerosis. Lancet Neurol 2010;9:599–612.
8. HLA-DRB1 - major histocompatibility complex, class II, DR beta 1. Bethesda (MD): U.S. National Library of Medicine; 2014. Web. 26 Jan. 2014. Available at: http://ghr.nlm.nih.gov/gene=HLA-DRB1.

9. Simpson S Jr, Blizzard L, Otahal P, et al. Latitude is significantly associated with the prevalence of Multiple Sclerosis: a meta-analysis. J Neurol Neurosurg Psychiatry 2011;82:1132–41.
10. Walsh N. Autoimmunity and a wily virus: is there a link? Autoimmunity and a wily virus: is there a link? MedPage Today 2014. Web. 26 Jan. 2014.
11. Hernan MA, Olek MJ, Ascherio A. Cigarette smoking and incidence of multiple sclerosis. Am J Epidemiol 2001;154:69–74.
12. Frohman EM, Racke MK, Raine CS. Multiple sclerosis: the plaque and its pathogenesis. N Engl J Med 2006;354:942–55.
13. Nylander A, Hafler DA. Multiple sclerosis. J Clin Invest 2012;122:1180–8.
14. Popescu BF, Pirko I, Lucchinetti CF. Pathology of multiple sclerosis: where do we stand? Continuum (Minneap Minn) 2013;19:901–21.
15. Goodin DS. Multiple sclerosis and other demyelinating diseases. Chapter 380. In: Longo DL, Fauci AS, Kasper DL, et al, editors. Harrison's principles of internal medicine. 18th edition. New York: McGraw-Hill; 2012. Available at: http://www.accessmedicine.com/content.aspx?aID=9147780. Accessed January 3, 2014.
16. Kurtzke JF. Rating neurological impairment in multiple sclerosis: an expanded disability scale. Neurology 1983;33:1444–52.
17. Marsha TL. Multiple Sclerosis Centers of Excellence. Kurtzke Expanded Disability Status Scale. Veterans Affairs Puget Sound Health Care System - Seattle, Dec 2009. Web. 01 Mar 2014.
18. Jelinek GA. Kurtzke EDSS scale. Overcoming multiple sclerosis. Overcoming MS; 2013. Web. 1 Jan. 2014.
19. Marcus JF, Waubant EL. Updates on clinically isolated syndrome and diagnostic criteria for multiple sclerosis. Neurohospitalist 2012;3(2):65–80.
20. Ali EN, Buckle GJ. Neuroimaging in multiple sclerosis. Neurol Clin 2009;27(1): 203–19.
21. Palace J. Making the diagnosis of multiple sclerosis. J Neurol Neurosurg Psychiatry 2001;71:ii3–8. Available at: http://www.ncbi.nlm.nih.gov/pmc/articles/PMC1765569/pdf/v071p00ii3.pdf.
22. Matloff J. Multiple sclerosis. Chapter 213. In: Matloff J, Dressler DD, Brotman DJ, et al, editors. Principles and practice of hospital medicine. New York: McGraw-Hill; 2012. Available at: http://www.accessmedicine.com/content.aspx?aID=56211606. Accessed January 3, 2014.
23. Miller DH, Weinshenker BG, Filippi M, et al. Differential diagnosis of suspected multiple sclerosis: a consensus approach. Mult Scler 2008;14:1157–74.
24. Marrie RA, Hanwell H. General health issues in multiple sclerosis: comorbidities, secondary conditions, and health behaviors. Continuum (Minneap Minn) 2013; 19(4):1046–57.
25. Blanco-Kelly F, Matesanz F, Alcina A, et al. CD40: novel association with Crohn's disease and replication in multiple sclerosis susceptibility. PLoS One 2010;5: e11520.
26. Eisenbarth GS. Banting Lecture 2009: An unfinished journey: molecular pathogenesis to prevention of type 1A diabetes. Diabetes 2010;59:759–74.
27. Rubin SM. Management of multiple sclerosis: an overview. Dis Mon 2013;59(7): 253–60.
28. Mullarkey C. FDA approves new treatment regimen for multiple sclerosis. Consultant 360; 2/11/14.
29. Polman CH, O'Connor PW, Havrdova E, et al. A randomized placebo-controlled trial of natalizumab for relapsing multiple sclerosis. N Engl J Med 2006;354(9): 899–910.

30. Bloomgren G, Richman S, Hotermans C, et al. Risk of natalizumab-associated progressive multifocal leukoencephalopathy. N Engl J Med 2012;366(20):1870–80.
31. Ransohoff R. Natalizumab for multiple sclerosis. N Engl J Med 2007;356(25):2622–9.
32. Pelletier D, Hafler DA. Fingolimod for multiple sclerosis. N Engl J Med 2012;366(4):339–47.
33. O'Connor P, Wolinsky JS, Confavreux C, et al. Randomized trial of teriflunomide for relapsing multiple sclerosis. N Engl J Med 2011;365(14):1293–303.
34. Fox RJ, Miller DH, Phillips JT, et al. Placebo-controlled phase 3 study of oral BG-12 or glatiramer in multiple sclerosis. N Engl J Med 2012;367(12):1087–97.
35. Calabresi P. Diagnosis and management of multiple sclerosis. Am Fam Physician 2004;70(10):1935–44.
36. Wening J, Ford J, Jouett LD. Orthotics and FES for maintenance of walking in patients with MS. Dis Mon 2013;59(8):284–9.

# Evaluation and Management of Amyotrophic Lateral Sclerosis

Nojan Valadi, MD

## KEYWORDS

- Amyotrophic lateral sclerosis (ALS) • Motor neuron disease (MND)
- Neurodegeneration • Diagnostic criteria • Neuromuscular disease

## KEY POINTS

- Consider amyotrophic lateral sclerosis (ALS) and motor neuron disease in patients who have upper and/or lower motor weakness without sensory problems (eg, extensor plantar responses plus atrophy and fasciculations).
- Consider ALS in patients with combined upper and lower motor neuron signs plus weakness in facial muscles.
- Obtain MRI of the brain and cervical spine, as well as electrodiagnostic and laboratory studies to exclude other diseases.
- Consider treatment options with supportive measures (multidisciplinary support to help cope with disability; drug treatment for symptoms such as spasticity, cramps, and pseudobulbar affect).

## INTRODUCTION

Amyotrophic lateral sclerosis (ALS) is a neurodegenerative motor neuron disease (MND) that results in progressive neuromuscular weakness. ALS, also known as "Lou Gehrig's disease," after the famous baseball player with the disorder, is the most common MND. Although most MNDs affect only the lower motor neurons, ALS can affect both upper motor neurons in the motor cortex in the brain and lower motor neurons in motor nuclei in the anterior horn of the spinal cord and the cranial nerve nuclei in the brainstem. Other MNDs are listed in **Table 1**, of which ALS is most common. The clinical presentation is typically one of atrophy, weakness, and fasciculations of muscles involved, all signs of lower motor neuron involvement

Disclosures: The author has no relationship with any commercial company that has a direct financial interest in the subject matter or materials discussed in the article.
St. Francis Neurology, 2300-A Manchester Expressway, Suite 201, Columbus, GA 31904, USA
E-mail address: nvaladi@gmail.com

Prim Care Clin Office Pract 42 (2015) 177–187
http://dx.doi.org/10.1016/j.pop.2015.01.009
0095-4543/15/$ – see front matter © 2015 Elsevier Inc. All rights reserved.
primarycare.theclinics.com

**Table 1**
**Motor neuron diseases**

| Motor Neuron Diseases | Upper Motor Neuron Involved | Lower Motor Neuron Involved |
|---|---|---|
| Amyotrophic lateral sclerosis | Yes | Yes |
| Primary lateral sclerosis | Yes | No |
| Progressive muscular atrophy | No | Yes |
| Progressive bulbar palsy | No | Yes |
| Spinal muscular atrophy | No | Yes |
| Spinobulbar muscular atrophy (Kennedy disease) | No | Yes |
| Poliomyelitis | No | Yes |
| Postpolio syndrome | No | Yes |
| Multifocal motor neuropathy | No | Yes |

together with involvement of cranial nerves that can cause speech and swallowing difficulties. The diagnosis is made based on clinical suspicion and confirmed with supportive testing. Imaging and genetic or infectious disease laboratory tests can either confirm or rule out specific differential diagnoses or mimics. Much can be done in supportive care for patients with ALS, but ALS is a progressive and fatal disease in which patients typically suffer respiratory failure. Treatment options at this time are very limited.

## EPIDEMIOLOGY
### Incidence and Prevalence

The incidence of ALS in Europe and North America is between 1.5 and 2.7 per 100,000 per year, with a prevalence of 2.7 to 7.4 per 100,000 and an overall lifetime risk of developing the disease of 1:400.[1,2] Men have a higher incidence (3.0 per 100,000 person-years; 95% confidence interval (CI) 2.8–3.3) than women (2.4 per 100,000 person-years; 95% CI 2.2–2.6), although the incidence between men and women is about the same in familial disease.[1] Roughly 20,000 Americans currently have ALS and another 5000 people are diagnosed with the disease annually. The disease onset peaks between ages 58 and 63 for sporadic ALS with a mean age of onset at 56, and that of familial ALS being approximately 10 years earlier.[1] Average disease duration from onset of symptoms is approximately 3 years, but it can vary significantly. ALS is familial in 5% to 10% and sporadic in 90% to 95% of cases.[3]

### Risk Factors and Genetics

Age and family history, as well as smoking, seem to be risk factors for the disease.[4,5] There are weak or conflicting data for other risk factors, including exposure to welding or soldering, exposure to heavy metal, military service, agricultural work, heavy manual labor, repetitive muscle use, work in the plastics industry, playing professional soccer, trauma, and electrical shock.[6–10]

Several genes have been identified in families with ALS and in some patients with sporadic ALS. These include mutations the *SOD1*, *FUS*, *OPTN*, *SETX*, *ANG*, *TARDBP*, *C9ORF72*, *SQSTM1*, and *ANG* genes.[11–19] *SOD1* accounts for 20% of familial ALS, causing a toxic gain of function with an autosomal dominant penetrance. Expansions in the *ATXN2* gene and duplications of the *SMN1* gene have also been shown to be associated with ALS, although interestingly not with familial ALS.[20–23] There is evidence suggesting several other low-risk genetic mutation sites that increase the susceptibility for sporadic ALS.[24]

Several western Pacific geographic locations have a higher than expected cluster of ALS. These include Guam, West New Guinea, and the Kii Peninsula in Japan. The ALS seen in these populations has a significant association with parkinsonism and has therefore been designated as amyotrophic lateral sclerosis–parkinsonism dementia complex (ALS-PDC).[25,26]

## Pathophysiology

The etiology of ALS is not well understood. The disease is characterized by motor neuron degeneration and death, with gliosis replacing neurons and causing a gradual and progressive loss of function. As the motor neuron undergoes apoptosis, the motor nerve axon degenerates, and the neuromuscular junction is destroyed. Muscle fibers innervated by that axon are denervated and subsequently atrophy. The individual fibers can be seen to have fibrillations and positive waves electrically, demonstrating muscle membrane instability. Fasciculations are seen when the fibers of a motor unit contract as a group. This can be seen both clinically and on electromyography (EMG). Adjacent motor nerve axons will initially reinnervate the muscle fibers (a recognizable pattern on EMG). With the eventual death of these motor neurons, the pattern of reinnervation abates and the predominating process of denervation is much more notable.[27,28] Muscle biopsy typically shows denervation atrophy together with fiber-type grouping, evidence of reinnervation. As cortical motor neurons are lost, retrograde axonal loss in the corticospinal tract leads to spinal cord atrophy. The ventral roots atrophy as large myelinated fibers are lost. Neuropathological examination can show degenerating neurons with intracellular inclusions.[29]

A number of mechanisms for the etiology of the death of motor neurons have been proposed, including abnormalities in RNA metabolism, *SOD1*-mediated toxicity, excitotoxicity, cytoskeletal derangements, mitochondrial dysfunction, viral infections, apoptosis, growth factor abnormalities, inflammatory responses, and others. Further research is pending at this time, but certainly it is believed that motor neuron cell death can be induced through multiple complex and variable mechanisms of genetic and acquired etiologies.

## Clinical Presentation and Diagnosis

Cellular death of motor neurons in ALS produces deficits affecting a limb, bulbar, axial, and respiratory function (**Table 2**). Depending on the limb, cranial nerve, or spinal cord segment affected, the disease can present uniquely initially, then progressing and spreading in variable ways to a typically invariable respiratory compromise. The initial clinical manifestation may be with upper motor neuron (UMN) or lower motor neuron (LMN) symptoms or signs (see **Table 2**), with the most common presentation at onset being asymmetric limb weakness, as seen in 80% of patients with ALS. Upper extremity weakness at onset is most common and typically involves the thenar hand muscles, with less effect on the hypothenar muscles.[30,31] Initially, ALS can affect the lower extremities by causing foot drop, and weakness of foot dorsiflexion distally and affecting the proximal muscles later in the disease course. Dysphagia or dysarthria can affect 20% of patients at onset of ALS affecting the brainstem. Patterns of onset also can include generalized weakness in the limbs or head and neck weakness, or weakness of paraspinal muscles, or respiratory muscle weakness, all of which are uncommon.[32,33]

**Table 2**
Upper motor neuron and lower motor neuron signs and symptoms of amyotrophic lateral sclerosis

| | Upper Motor Neuron Signs/ Symptoms | Lower Motor Neuron Signs/ Symptoms |
|---|---|---|
| Limbs | Spasticity, increased reflexes, Hoffman sign, upping toe, clonus, spastic and stiff gait, slowness, fine motor coordination difficulty, difficulty writing, falls, poor balance, difficulty with activities of daily living | Weakness in hands or feet, atrophy of hand muscles, foot drop, difficulty standing from chair or floor, fasciculations, difficulty climbing stairs, cramping, reduced reflexes |
| Bulbar | Jaw spasticity, increased jaw reflex, palmomental sign, slow tongue movement, trismus, jaw clonus, dysarthria, dysphagia, laryngospasms, pseudobulbar affect with inappropriate laughter and crying, drooling, | Tongue weakness, facial diplegia, jaw weakness, eye lid lag, dysphagia, dysarthria, tongue fasciculations, hoarseness, poor lip closure, difficulty chewing, dysarthria |
| Axial | Absent abdominal reflexes, spasticity and imbalance | Neck or truncal extension weakness, difficulty holding head up or standing upright, abdominal protuberance |
| Respiratory | | Tachypnea, hypophonia, use of accessory muscles, weak cough, morning headache, hallucinations, confusion |

When after initial presentation of symptoms, the disease progresses to include both UMN and LMN symptoms and signs and spreads to other segments over months to years, the diagnosis of ALS is confirmed. The progressive course is not one that is relapsing and remitting, but simply progresses without any return of function or improvement. Muscle wasting and weight loss, despite normal nutritional intake, also can occur. Absence of associated neuropathic or radiculopathic pain, sensory loss, sphincter dysfunction, ptosis, or extraocular nerve or muscle dysfunction also suggest and support the diagnosis of ALS. Although 20% to 30% of patients may have sensory symptoms, typically the sensory examination is normal.[32,34]

When tremor, dyskinesias, or supranuclear gaze paresis or autonomic dysfunction is seen, typically ALS can be excluded. However some of these features have been seen as part of an ALS-PLUS syndrome.[35] Patients with ALS can have cognitive dysfunction in 40% to 50% of cases. Frontotemporal type of executive dysfunction is what is typically seen; however, usually detectable only with formal cognitive testing. The *TARDBP* gene mutation that has been identified that leads to accumulation of TDP-43 protein in cytoplasmic inclusions in frontotemporal dementia also are seen in ALS and may explain some of the comorbidity of this type of cognitive dysfunction in ALS. This overlap between the 2 diseases is becoming increasingly evident clinically as well as molecularly.[36] It is therefore important to inquire about family history of dementia as well as MND in addition to Parkinson disease.[29]

## PHYSICAL EXAMINATION

The neurologic examination in the diagnosis of ALS, together with the revised El Escorial criteria, are key to clinching the diagnosis of ALS.[37] As ALS affects motor neurons affecting limb, bulbar, axial, and respiratory functions (see **Table 2**), the progressive nature of these symptoms with spread to other segments categorizes the disease. LMN findings include weakness, atrophy, and fasciculations. UMN findings include increased tone, spasticity, and increased deep tendon reflexes (**Table 3**). The examination should focus on identifying and characterizing the patterns of weakness and atrophy, while spending several minutes examining the entire body surface observing closely to identify fasciculations. Of equal importance is determining the presence of reflexes in muscles that are profoundly weak and wasted, pathologic reflexes such as crossed adductors, an upping toe or Babinski sign (toe extension in response to plantar stimulation), a jaw jerk, Tromner sign, Hoffman sign, or triple flexion of the lower extremities. Physical examination also certainly seeks to rule out reversible or treatable causes of the symptoms. If cranial nerves are affected and findings are consistent with ALS however, a treatable alternative cause is less likely.

## DIAGNOSTIC TESTING

EMG and nerve conduction studies (NCS/NCV), as well as MRI imaging of the brain and spinal cord, are required diagnostic tests to rule out potential other causes of the patient's symptoms. EMG can show both active denervation (fibrillations, positive waves) and reinnervation (reduced numbers of large-amplitude, long-duration, polyphasic motor unit potentials) in affected muscles.[27,28] EMG must be performed in at least 3 regions to rule out a localized polyradiculopathy or motor neuropathy and rather a more widespread process.

Laboratory tests should be performed to rule out other diseases, such as neuromuscular transmission disorders, myopathies, spinal muscular atrophies, polymyositis, dermatomyositis, thyroid and adrenal disorders, electrolyte abnormalities, infections such as syphilis, Lyme disease, hepatitis C, HIV, or other autoimmune-mediated motor neuropathies such as chronic inflammatory demyelinating polyneuropathy or of paraneoplastic etiology. A lumbar puncture can be performed if indicated and cerebrospinal fluid analysis can reveal an elevation in white blood cells or protein level, thereby suggesting an alternate diagnosis. Genetic testing (*SOD1* mutation or genetic abnormalities that cause spinal muscular atrophies) can be done if suggested by history, but only after the patient is counseled in this regard.

## DIAGNOSTIC CRITERIA

The revised El Escorial World Federation of Neurology criteria (**Fig. 1**) outline the clinical standard for the diagnosis of ALS.[37] These criteria, developed for appropriate enrollment of patients for research trials, help assign a degree of certainty to the

| Table 3 | | |
|---------|---|---|
| Simplified review of the difference between upper motor neuron and lower motor neuron findings | | |
| **Upper Motor Neuron vs Lower Motor Neuron Lesions** | | |
| | **Upper Motor Neuron Lesion** | **Lower Motor Neuron Lesion** |
| Reflexes | Increased | Diminished/Absent |
| Tone | Increased | Diminished/Absent |
| Bulk | Normal/Atrophied | Atrophied |
| Fasciculations | Absent | Present |

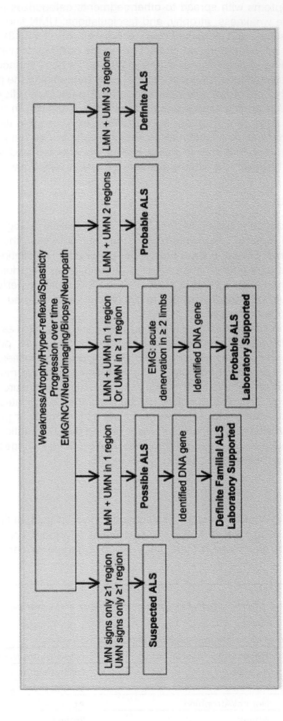

**Fig. 1.** El Escorial World Federation of Neurology criteria for diagnosis of ALS. (*From* Brooks BR, Miller RG, Swash M, et al. El Escorial revisited: revised criteria for the diagnosis of amyotrophic lateral sclerosis. Amyotroph Lateral Scler Other Motor Neuron Disord 2000;1:295; with permission.)

diagnosis and have been validated pathologically for their sensitivity and specificity.[38] The diagnosis of ALS by these criteria requires the following:

- Evidence of LMN disease by clinical, electrophysiological, or neuropathological examination
- Evidence of UMN disease degeneration by clinical examination
- Progressive spread of symptoms or signs within a region or to other regions, as determined by history or examination

More up-to-date Awaji criteria were proposed in 2008, allowing the addition of electrodiagnostic criteria (fasciculation potentials) for LMN signs to be used in conjunction to determine if a single limb is affected.[39] The Awaji criteria had a higher sensitivity compared with the revised El Escorial criteria (81% vs 62%), with equal specificity of 98%.[40]

Other MNDs, variants of ALS, and ALS mimics (also see **Table 1**) include the following:

- Progressive muscular atrophy: present with only progressive LMN findings that never involve UMNs. However at autopsy, they are found to have UMN pathology, including corticospinal tract abnormalities and motor cortex TDP-43 inclusions.[41,42]
- Primary lateral sclerosis: present with only UMN disease and never progress to involve LMNs clinically or electrodiagnostically.[43]
- Progressive bulbar palsy: UMN and LMN disease of the cranial nerves that typically progresses to bulbar-onset ALS.[44]
- Flail arm syndrome (brachial amyotrophic diplegia): progressive LMN atrophy and weakness affecting the proximal arm and spreading distally to the hand.[45]
- Flail leg syndrome (pseudopolyneuritic variant of ALS/MND): characterized by progressive LMN atrophy and weakness in the distal leg that eventually progresses to involve other regions, but much more slowly than classic ALS.[45]
- ALS-plus syndrome: classic symptoms of ALS along with features of other disorders, such as frontotemporal dementia, supranuclear gaze paresis, sensory loss, autonomic insufficiency, or parkinsonism.[35]
- Multifocal motor neuropathy: a demyelinating LMN disease that affects one limb progressing to other limbs, with weakness out of proportion to atrophy, without UMN involvement. Anti-GM1 antibodies are often seen.[46]
- Spinal muscular atrophy: a variable lower MND with a genetic mutation of the *SMN1* gene, with Type IV of the disease presenting in adulthood with proximal leg weakness that does not progress or affect life expectancy.[47]
- Spinal bulbar muscular atrophy (Kennedy disease): Adult-onset X-linked trinucleotide CAG repeat causing MND with men always affected, and presenting in the fourth to seventh decades with bulbar-onset LMN disease, diabetes, gynecomastia, and impotence, with slowly progressive neuromuscular symptoms.[48]

## DISEASE COURSE AND MANAGEMENT

As the disease progresses and spreads to other segments, the patient's weakness advances and burden of disability accrues. The patient goes through various emotional and clinical stages of the disease. Patients and families need help coping with progressive disability and loss of function as well as making end-of-life plans. A team-based approach involving the patient, the caregiver, and the physician can help patients understand, deal with, and make many of these hard decisions, including planning for hospice care and death. Multidisciplinary approaches to ALS patient care can help facilitate quality of life, improve outcomes, prognosis, and decrease need for emergency care.[49] In these settings, monitoring functional impairment and disease progression is an integral part of the monitoring and management of the patient with ALS. The Revised ALS Functional Rating Scale is currently the most widely used assessment tool; scores are used to predict survival, and have been used extensively in clinical trials.[50]

Riluzole, the only drug approved by the Food and Drug Administration for treatment of ALS, remains the only effective drug, and extends the average survival of patients by 3 to 6 months. Riluzole blocks the release of glutamate and is thought to decrease neuronal excitotoxicity.[51,52] Liver enzymes need to be monitored closely if the patient is started on riluzole. Optimal treatment is based on symptom management, supportive care, and preservation of quality of life, provided in a multidisciplinary setting. Death is usually caused by respiratory failure, with median mortality of 3 years of onset. Five-year and 10-year survival are 20% and 10%, respectively. Survival for more than 30 years is rare. In progressive bulbar palsy with ALS (bulbar-variant ALS), deterioration and death occur more rapidly.

The following are interventions to help symptoms in ALS:

- For spasticity: stretching, tizanidine, baclofen, clonazepam, or botulinum toxin
- For cramps: stretching, massage, magnesium oxide, vitamin E, carbamazepine, quinine, or phenytoin
- To decrease saliva production: a home suction device, anticholinergic drugs (glycopyrrolate, amitriptyline, benztropine, trihexyphenidyl, transdermal hyoscine, atropine)
- For pseudobulbar affect: dextromethorphan, amitriptyline, fluvoxamine, selective serotonin reuptake inhibitors
- For pain: stretching, massage, acupuncture, nonsteroidal anti-inflammatory drugs, acetaminophen, or morphine sulfate
- For laryngospasms: lorazepam, proton pump inhibitor
- For insomnia: sleep hygiene, amitriptyline, trazodone, chloral hydrate, diphenhydramine
- For fatigue: amantadine, methylphenidate
- For early satiety: metoclopramide before meals
- For air hunger: meditation, breathing exercises, lorazepam, morphine sulfate

Patients with ALS who have difficulty speaking may benefit from working with a speech therapist. A coordinated approach by the primary care physician and neurologist is necessary with a focus on treatment options, durable medical equipment needs, and end-of-life discussions. Multidisciplinary approaches that involve a spectrum of care providers, as outlined later in this article, have had the most success in optimizing patient care, satisfaction, and outcomes.[49] Evaluation by speech therapists, physical therapists, respiratory therapists, and occupational therapists, as well as meeting with social workers and hospice nurses during the patient's multidisciplinary visit, can help improve outcome and meet all of the patient's needs. These could include special equipment or devices, such as ramps, braces, walkers, and wheelchairs, that can help patients with ALS keep their independence and remain mobile.

Pulmonary function evaluations are typically done during visits to assess for a need for ventilator support. The forced vital capacity (FVC) is a good measure of respiratory function in ALS and a decreased of FVC to less than 50% of predicted is associated with respiratory symptoms. When the FVC decreases to 25% to 30% of predicted, the patient has a significant risk of respiratory failure or sudden death. Physicians should monitor FVC and have end-of-life conversations with patients before FVC decreases to less than 50% or patients develop nocturnal hypoventilation or dyspnea.[53]

Speech therapists help in the evaluation of swallowing and a need for nutritional support via feeding tube to help reduce the risk of choking and pneumonia. Social workers, hospice nurses, and home care specialists can help patients and their families with the medical, emotional, and financial challenges of coping with ALS, especially during the final stages.

## SUMMARY

ALS is the most common MND, presenting with progressive LMN and UMN deficits. Although neuroimaging, laboratory tests, and EMG are performed to rule out ALS mimics, the physical examination is the key to the diagnosis of ALS. Treatment is dependent on the etiology, but MNDs are not reversible. A coordinated approach by the primary care physician and neurologist with a focus on multidisciplinary care is necessary to optimize quality of life and meet the patient's needs.

## REFERENCES

1. Worms PM. The epidemiology of motor neuron diseases: a review of recent studies. J Neurol Sci 2001;191:3.
2. Logroscino G, Traynor BJ, Hardiman O, et al. Incidence of amyotrophic lateral sclerosis in Europe. J Neurol Neurosurg Psychiatry 2010;81:385.
3. Byrne S, Walsh C, Lynch C, et al. Rate of familial amyotrophic lateral sclerosis: a systematic review and meta-analysis. J Neurol Neurosurg Psychiatry 2011; 82:623.
4. Sutedja NA, Veldink JH, Fischer K, et al. Lifetime occupation, education, smoking, and risk of ALS. Neurology 2007;69:1508.
5. Armon C. Smoking may be considered an established risk factor for sporadic ALS. Neurology 2009;73:1693.
6. Armon C, Kurland LT, Daube JR, et al. Epidemiologic correlates of sporadic amyotrophic lateral sclerosis. Neurology 1991;41:1077.
7. Chiò A, Benzi G, Dossena M, et al. Severely increased risk of amyotrophic lateral sclerosis among Italian professional football players. Brain 2005;128:472.
8. Felmus MT, Patten BM, Swanke L. Antecedent events in amyotrophic lateral sclerosis. Neurology 1976;26:167.
9. Rowland LP, Shneider NA. Amyotrophic lateral sclerosis. N Engl J Med 2001; 344:1688.
10. Weisskopf MG, O'Reilly EJ, McCullough ML, et al. Prospective study of military service and mortality from ALS. Neurology 2005;64:32.
11. Gellera C, Castellotti B, Riggio MC, et al. Superoxide dismutase gene mutations in Italian patients with familial and sporadic amyotrophic lateral sclerosis: identification of three novel missense mutations. Neuromuscul Disord 2001;11:404.
12. Greenway MJ, Andersen PM, Russ C, et al. ANG mutations segregate with familial and 'sporadic' amyotrophic lateral sclerosis. Nat Genet 2006;38:411.
13. Sreedharan J, Blair IP, Tripathi VB, et al. TDP-43 mutations in familial and sporadic amyotrophic lateral sclerosis. Science 2008;319:1668.
14. Talbot K. Another gene for ALS: mutations in sporadic cases and the rare variant hypothesis. Neurology 2009;73:1172.
15. Belzil VV, Valdmanis PN, Dion PA, et al. Mutations in FUS cause FALS and SALS in French and French Canadian populations. Neurology 2009;73:1176.

16. Lattante S, Conte A, Zollino M, et al. Contribution of major amyotrophic lateral sclerosis genes to the etiology of sporadic disease. Neurology 2012;79:66.
17. Zhao ZH, Chen WZ, Wu ZY, et al. A novel mutation in the senataxin gene identified in a Chinese patient with sporadic amyotrophic lateral sclerosis. Amyotroph Lateral Scler 2009;10:118.
18. Rubino E, Rainero I, Chiò A, et al. SQSTM1 mutations in frontotemporal lobar degeneration and amyotrophic lateral sclerosis. Neurology 2012;79:1556.
19. Teyssou E, Takeda T, Lebon V, et al. Mutations in SQSTM1 encoding p62 in amyotrophic lateral sclerosis: genetics and neuropathology. Acta Neuropathol 2013;125:511.
20. Van Damme P, Veldink JH, van Blitterswijk M, et al. Expanded ATXN2 CAG repeat size in ALS identifies genetic overlap between ALS and SCA2. Neurology 2011; 76:2066.
21. Sorarù G, Clementi M, Forzan M, et al. ALS risk but not phenotype is affected by ataxin-2 intermediate length polyglutamine expansion. Neurology 2011;76:2030.
22. Fischbeck KH, Pulst SM. Amyotrophic lateral sclerosis and spinocerebellar ataxia 2. Neurology 2011;76:2050.
23. Blauw HM, Barnes CP, van Vught PW, et al. SMN1 gene duplications are associated with sporadic ALS. Neurology 2012;78:776.
24. Traynor BJ, Singleton A. Genome-wide association studies and ALS: are we there yet? Lancet Neurol 2007;6:841.
25. Zimmerman HM. Monthly report to the medical officer in command. Dayton (OH): United States Navy; Medical Research Unit No. 2. 1945.
26. Curled LT, Mulder DW. Epidemiologic investigations of amyotrophic lateral sclerosis. I. Preliminary report on geographic distribution, with special reference to the Mariana Islands, including clinical and pathologic observations. Neurology 1954;4:355.
27. Daube JR. Electrodiagnostic studies in amyotrophic lateral sclerosis and other motor neuron disorders. Muscle Nerve 2000;23:1488.
28. Krivickas LS. Amyotrophic lateral sclerosis and other motor neuron diseases. Phys Med Rehabil Clin N Am 2003;14:327.
29. Giordana MT, Ferrero P, Grifoni S, et al. Dementia and cognitive impairment in ALS: a review. Neurol Sci 2011;32(1):9–16.
30. Wilbourn AJ. The "split hand syndrome". Muscle Nerve 2000;23:138.
31. Kuwabara S, Sonoo M, Komori T, et al. Dissociated small hand muscle atrophy in amyotrophic lateral sclerosis: frequency, extent, and specificity. Muscle Nerve 2008;37:426.
32. Mitsumoto H, Chad D, Pioro EP. Monograph. Amyotrophic lateral sclerosis. Contemporary Neurology Series 49. Philadelphia: F. A. Davis. 1997. p. 1–480.
33. Shoesmith CL, Findlater K, Rowe A, et al. Prognosis of amyotrophic lateral sclerosis with respiratory onset. J Neurol Neurosurg Psychiatry 2007;78:629.
34. Hammad M, Silva A, Glass J, et al. Clinical, electrophysiologic, and pathologic evidence for sensory abnormalities in ALS. Neurology 2007;69:2236.
35. McCluskey LF, Elman LB, Martinez-Lage M, et al. Amyotrophic lateral sclerosis-plus syndrome with TAR DNA-binding protein-43 pathology. Arch Neurol 2009;66:121.
36. Turner MR, Hardiman O, Benatar M, et al. Controversies and priorities in amyotrophic lateral sclerosis. Lancet Neurol 2013;12:310.
37. Brooks BR, Miller RG, Swash M, et al. El Escorial revisited: revised criteria for the diagnosis of amyotrophic lateral sclerosis. Amyotroph Lateral Scler Other Mot Neuron Disord 2000;1:293.

38. Chaudhuri KR, Crump S, al-Sarraj S, et al. The validation of El Escorial criteria for the diagnosis of amyotrophic lateral sclerosis: a clinicopathological study. J Neurol Sci 1995;129(Suppl):11.
39. de Carvalho M, Dengler R, Eisen A, et al. Electrodiagnostic criteria for diagnosis of ALS. Clin Neurophysiol 2008;119:497.
40. Costa J, Swash M, de Carvalho M. Awaji criteria for the diagnosis of amyotrophic lateral sclerosis: a systematic review. Arch Neurol 2012;69:1410.
41. Ince PG, Evans J, Knopp M, et al. Corticospinal tract degeneration in the progressive muscular atrophy variant of ALS. Neurology 2003;60:1252.
42. Tsuchiya K, Sano M, Shiotsu H, et al. Sporadic amyotrophic lateral sclerosis of long duration mimicking spinal progressive muscular atrophy exists: additional autopsy case with a clinical course of 19 years. Neuropathology 2004;24:228.
43. Singer MA, Statland JM, Wolfe GI, et al. Primary lateral sclerosis. Muscle Nerve 2007;35:291.
44. Donaghy M. Classification and clinical features of motor neuron diseases and motor neuropathies in adults. J Neurol 1999;246:331.
45. Wijesekera LC, Mathers S, Talman P, et al. Natural history and clinical features of the flail arm and flail leg ALS variants. Neurology 2009;72:1087.
46. Muley SA, Parry GJ. Multifocal motor neuropathy. J Clin Neurosci 2012;19:1201.
47. Zerres K, Rudnik-Schöneborn S, Forkert R, et al. Genetic basis of adult-onset spinal muscular atrophy. Lancet 1995;346:1162.
48. Finsterer J. Perspectives of Kennedy's disease. J Neurol Sci 2010;298:1.
49. Traynor BJ, Alexander M, Corr B, et al. Effect of a multidisciplinary amyotrophic lateral sclerosis (ALS) clinic on ALS survival: a population based study, 1996-2000. J Neurol Neurosurg Psychiatry 2003;74(9):1258–61.
50. Cedarbaum JM, Stambler N, Malta E, et al. The ALSFRS-R: a revised ALS functional rating scale that incorporates assessments of respiratory function. J Neurol Sci 1999;169(1–2):13–21.
51. Traynor BJ, Alexander M, Corr B, et al. An outcome study of riluzole in amyotrophic lateral sclerosis—a population-based study in Ireland, 1996–2000. J Neurol 2003;250(4):473–9.
52. Zoccolella S, Beghi E, Palagano G, et al. Riluzole and amyotrophic lateral sclerosis survival: a population-based study in southern Italy. Eur J Neurol 2007; 14(3):262–8.
53. Rabinstein AA, Wijdicks EF. Warning signs of imminent respiratory failure in neurological patients. Semin Neurol 2003;23:97.

# Guillain-Barré Syndrome

Vibhuti Ansar, MD[a],*, Nojan Valadi, MD[b]

## KEYWORDS

- Guillain-Barré syndrome • Demyelinating syndrome
- Acute inflammatory demyelinating polyradiculoneuropathy (AIDP)
- Acute motor axonal neuropathy • Miller Fisher syndrome

## KEY POINTS

- Guillain-Barré syndrome (GBS) has several clinical variants, including acute inflammatory demyelinating polyradiculoneuropathy (AIDP), acute motor axonal neuropathy, acute motor and sensory axonal neuropathy, acute pandysautonomia, sensory GBS, GBS with ophthalmoplegia, and Miller Fisher syndrome.
- The incidence typically is 1 to 2 per 100,000, with a higher prevalence in men and the elderly.
- GBS is often preceded by an acute viral infection and has been linked to vaccine administration.
- Treatment may consist of several cycles of plasma exchange (PE) or intravenous immunoglobulin (IVIG). Both treatments are effective. Corticosteroids have not been shown to help in GBS.
- Approximately 80% to 90% of patients recover with no sequelae at 1 year.

## INTRODUCTION

Acquired inflammatory demyelinating polyradiculoneuropathies are immunologically mediated and can be classified by their clinical time course as acute or chronic or by the constellation of symptoms and electrophysiologic pattern into one of several GBS variants. In AIDP, the most common type of GBS, the maximal deficits appear over days (at most 4 weeks), followed by a plateau phase and then gradual improvement, whereas chronic inflammatory demyelinating polyradiculoneuropathy may be more slowly progressive or relapsing. The axonal variants of GBS may be purely motor or both sensory and motor neuropathies, both of which can be severe with poor recovery. The clinical features of GBS as described by Guillan, Barré, and Strohl in 1916, were motor weakness, areflexia, paresthesias with slight sensory loss, and cerebrospinal fluid (CSF) albuminocytologic dissociation. GBS has several clinical variants,

[a] Department of Medical Education, Midtown Medical Center, Columbus Regional Healthcare, 1900 10th Avenue, Suite 100, Columbus, GA 31901, USA; [b] 2300-A Manchester Expressway, Suite 201, Columbus, GA 31903, USA
* Corresponding author.
E-mail address: vibhuti.ansar@columbusregional.com

Prim Care Clin Office Pract 42 (2015) 189–193
http://dx.doi.org/10.1016/j.pop.2015.01.001
0095-4543/15/$ – see front matter © 2015 Elsevier Inc. All rights reserved.

including acute motor axonal neuropathy, acute motor and sensory axonal neuropathy, and Miller Fisher syndrome.[1] The subtypes differ in pathologic and electrodiagnostic features. Some clinical distinctions are also present, especially with Miller Fisher variant.[2]

## EPIDEMIOLOGY

With the decline of acute poliomyelitis, GBS has become the most common acute paralytic disease in Western countries. Incidence of GBS is approximately 1 to 2 per 100,000 and afflicts men and the elderly more commonly than women or younger patients.[3]

## RISK FACTORS

GBS is typically preceded by an infection, most frequently from an upper respiratory tract (58%) or gastrointestinal source (22%), but may also be caused by surgery or being immunized 1 to 4 weeks prior to the onset of symptoms.[4] Campylobacter jejuni is the most commonly identified bacteria associated with the acute motor axonal neuropathy and GBS variants. Immunizations that have been linked to the development of GBS include swine flu, tetanus, diphtheria toxoids as well as rabies.[3] Several viral infections (cytomegalovirus, Epstein-Barr virus, HIV, varicella-zoster virus, and hepatitis A and B); drugs, such as heroin, suramin, and streptokinase; and chronic conditions (like systemic lupus erythematosus and HIV) have predisposed to GBS patients.

## CLINICAL FEATURES

GBS and variants typically present with progressively ascending fairly symmetric paralysis and areflexia over the course of hours to several days. Motor paralysis affects the lower extremities more frequently than the upper extremeties.[5] Sensory disturbances may or may not occur. Respiratory failure due to neuromuscular compromise is not uncommon, often requiring supportive ventilation.[6] Autonomic symptoms have been reported in as many as 65% of patients admitted to hospitals for GBS and may include orthostatic hypotension, anhidrosis, urinary retention, gastrointestinal atony, or iridoplegia.[7] Miller Fisher syndrome, which accounts for 5% of GBS cases, is characterized by ophthalmoplegia, ataxia, and areflexia. Patients present with diplopia followed by discoordination of the limbs and gait. **Tables 1** and **2** indicate various physical signs and symptoms in patients with GBS.

## DIAGNOSIS

Several consensus statements have been made about the required diagnostic criteria for GBS and variants. Required criteria for the diagnosis include progressive weakness of more than 2 limbs, areflexia, and progression for no more than 4 weeks.[3] Supportive criteria include mild sensory signs, relative symmetry of symptoms, absence of fever, facial diplegia, and a cerebrospinal fluid (CSF) profile of albuminocytologic dissociation with elevated protein concentration without CSF pleocytosis, with the exception of the setting of HIV, where pleocytosis is the norm and not the exception.[8] Laboratory testing could show an elevated erythrocyte sedimentation rate, mildly abnormal renal and liver laboratory results, and electrolyte disturbances, such as hyponatremia (from the syndrome of inappropriate secretion of antidiuretic hormone). Nerve conduction studies may be abnormal and show slowed motor conduction velocities, partial conduction block, and dispersed motor responses. Demyelination at the nerve roots may cause absent or delayed F-wave responses or H-reflexes on the studies. MRI of the lumbosacral spine typically shows enhancement of the nerve

**Table 1**
**Percentage of patients with these physical signs in GBS**

| | |
|---|---|
| Flaccid weakness | 100% |
| Limb areflexia/hyporeflexia | 100% |
| Distal weakness (predominant) | 33.3% |
| Distal sensory loss | 38.9% |
| Cranial nerve VII palsy | 31.5% |
| Proximal weakness (predominant) | 27.8% |
| Palate paralysis | 14.8% |
| Respiratory failure requiring ICU | 14.8% |
| Fluctuating arterial HTN | 9.3% |
| Papilledema | 7.4% |
| Ocular nerve palsy | 5.6% |
| Weakness of jaw | 3.7% |

*Data from* Bahemuka M. Guillain-Barre syndrome in Kenya: a clinical review of 54 patients. J Neurol 1988;235:418–21.

roots.[9] This inflammatory response at the nerve roots helps explain certain features, including the CSF findings, some neurophysiologic findings, and autonomic dysfunction that may be seen in these patients. In Miller Fisher syndrome, serum IgG antibodies to ganglioside GQ1b are found in most patients.

## THERAPEUTIC OPTIONS

PE and IVIG are common treatments for GBS. Combination therapy is not superior to either alone. Both are expensive but decrease the time to recovery.[3] Both treatment modalities are superior to supportive therapy alone. No significant differences have been found between the two treatment options for disability scores at 4 weeks or the time to wean ventilatory support or recover unassisted walking.[10] Patients receiving IVIG, however, have fewer side effects, have fewer complications, and are less likely to quit therapy compared with those receiving PE.[11]

PE involves taking the autoantibodies out of the blood. It cannot be performed in pregnant patients or hemodynamically unstable patients. Practice guidelines set by

**Table 2**
**Presenting symptoms**

| | |
|---|---|
| Limb weakness | 100% |
| Numbness/paresthesias | 60% |
| Difficulty breathing | 34% |
| Choking | 20.4% |
| Sphincter disturbance | 18.5% |
| Slurring speech | 11.1% |
| Double vision | 7.4% |
| Headache | 5.6% |
| Difficulty chewing | 3.7% |

*Data from* Bahemuka M. Guillain-Barre syndrome in Kenya: a clinical review of 54 patients. J Neurol 1988;235:418–21.

the Quality Standards Subcommittee of the American Academy of Neurology (AAN) in 2003 endorse the use of PE within 4 weeks of symptom onset in nonambulatory patients and 2 weeks in ambulatory patients. Common side effects include hypotension, hypocalcemia, and thrombocytopenia (typically improves within 24–48 hours). If patients need to undergo multiple exchanges, episodes should occur 24 hours apart to help avoid the decrease in hemostatic factors: 2 to 6 treatments in a 1- to 2-week period have been shown effective.[2,12] Each session should exchange plasma volume (50 mL/kg) with albumin (preferred over fresh frozen plasma). Long-term benefits from PE therapy include recovered muscle strength, lower likelihood of motor dysfunction, and fewer relapses at 1 year compared with supportive care.[12]

IVIG preparations differ depending on the manufacturer, with varying osmolality, salt and sugar content, pH, and IgA content. Treatment with IVIG must be judiciously individualized. The main component of IVIG is IgG. The usual dose is 2 g/kg divided over 2 to 5 days. High-dose IVIG has not been shown to be superior to low-dose IVIG. Vital signs should be checked every 15 minutes during the first hour and then periodically after. Acetaminophen or an antihistamine may be given prior to each dose. Renal function should be tested prior to each dose and periodically after. A repeat course may be given if there is an inadequate response. People with renal dysfunction should have the rate of infusion halved of the normal rate. Serious adverse side effects include venous throembolism, anaphylaxis, acute renal failure, aseptic meningitis, and stroke-like episodes.[11] Due to the risk of anaphylaxis in patients with IgA deficiency due to anti-IgA antibodies, IgA levels should be tested prior to administration of IVIG.[12] The Quality Standards Subcommittee of the AAN endorses starting IVIG therapy within 2 to 4 weeks of disease onset in people unable to walk without assistance.

Corticosteroids are not beneficial in GBS. Corticosteroids in combination with IVIG or alone have not shown benefit in a Cochrane review. Some studies showed steroids delayed recovery. The time to recovery of unaided walking, time to discontinuation of ventilation, and death rates were no better in the corticosteroid group compared with placebo. Relapse rates did not differ. Diabetes developed in the steroid group more frequently than with placebo. Hypertension (HTN) occurred less frequently in intravenous steroid studies, however.[13]

Supportive care is essential in the treatment of GBS. Prophylaxis for deep vein thrombosis using heparin, enoxaparin, or support stockings until patients can ambulate independently is vital. Respiratory function and pulse/blood pressure monitoring should occur in GBS patients but not enough evidence exists to suggest specific methods. Tracheostomy should be performed after 2 weeks in patients whose respiratory status has not improved. Simple analgesics like acetaminophen and nonsteroidal anti-inflammatory drugs may not be effective. Opioid analgesics improve pain but must be monitored for side effects secondary to autonomic denervation (gut dysmotility and bladder distention). Adjuvant therapy with tricyclic antidepressants, tramadol, gabapentin, and carbamazepine may aid GBS. Monitoring bowel and bladder function should occur daily and rehabilitation therapy should focus on proper limb positioning, posture, orthotics, and nutrition. Immunizations should not be given in the acute phase or for 1 year after a GBS episode. Thereafter, immunizations should not be withheld unless there is a concern that one caused the disease. If so, only that particular immunization should be withheld.[6]

## CLINICAL OUTCOMES

Overall, patients afflicted with GBS have a good prognosis. Improvements in critical care have vastly changed outcomes from GBS, decreasing mortality from 33% to

5% to 10% with the introduction of positive pressure ventilation. A great majority of patients recover with minimal deficits at 1 year.[5] Some patients have persistent disabilities.[10]

## SUMMARY

In conclusion, GBS and its clinical variants are a group of rapidly progressing, potentially debilitating neurologic disorders that may have significant morbidity/mortality if left unrecognized or untreated. The most common symptoms include ascending limb weakness and paralysis, which may progress to respiratory failure. Diagnosis is made clinically with laboratory testing. Several treatment options exist, including PE and IVIG administration. Most cases may resolve without sequelae, but those that do not may leave behind significant persistent debility.

## REFERENCES

1. Beghi E, Kurland LT, Mulder DW, et al. Guiilan-Barre syndrome: clinicoepidemiologic features and effects of influenza vaccine. Arch Neurol 1985;42:1053–7.
2. Asbury AK. New concepts of Guillain-Barre syndrome. J Child Neurol 2000;15: 183–91.
3. Winer JB. Guillain-Barre syndrome. Mol Pathol 2001;54:381–5.
4. Govoni V, Granieri E. Epidemiology of the Guillain-Barre syndrome. Curr Opin Neurol 2001;14:605–13.
5. Gonzalez-Suarez I, Sanz-Gallego I, Rodríguez de Rivera FJ, et al. Guillain-Barre syndrome: natural history and prognostic factors: a retrospective review of 106 cases. BMC Neurol 2013;13:95.
6. Hughes R, Wijdicks EF, Benson E, et al. Supportive care for patients with Guillain-Barre snydrome. Arch Neurol 2005;62:1194–8.
7. Zochodne DW. Autonomic involvement in Guillain-Barre syndrome: a review. Muscle Nerve 1994;17:1145–55.
8. Asbury AK, Cornblath DR. Assessment of current diagnostic criteria for Guillain-Barré syndrome. Ann Neurol 1990;27(Suppl):S21–4.
9. Bertorini T, Halford H, Lawrence J, et al. Contrast-enhanced magnetic resonance imaging of the lumbosacral roots in the dysimmune inflammatory poluneuropathies. J Neuroimaging 1995;5:9–15.
10. Hughes RA, Swan AV, Cornblath DR, et al. Randomised trial of plasma exchange, intravenous immunoglobulin, and combined treatments in Guillain-Barre syndrome. Lancet 1997;349:225–30.
11. Cochrane Collaboration. IVIg for GBS. 2012.
12. Sederholm BH. Treatment of acute immune-medicated neuropathies: Guillain-Barre syndrome and clinical variants. Semin Neurol 2010;30(4):365–72.
13. Hughes RA, van Doorn PA. Corticosteroids for Guillain-Barre syndrome. Cochrane Database Syst Rev 2012;(8):CD001446.

# A Practical Approach to Dementia in the Outpatient Primary Care Setting

CrossMark

Mark D. Darrow, MD

## KEYWORDS

- Dementia • Diagnosis • Treatment • Primary care

## KEY POINTS

- The work-up and treatment of most dementias can be accomplished in a primary care outpatient setting.
- Treatment options should begin with nonpharmacologic interventions.
- Pharmacologic treatment should be focused, be prescribed for a period of time, and have treatment goals in mind.
- Frequent office visits help to address patient and family concerns and reinforce treatment goals.
- A multidisciplinary approach to the care of dementia patients can be achieved in any community with the right knowledge of available services.

## INTRODUCTION

The diagnosis of dementia is among the most feared and one of the commonly encountered diseases in a primary care setting. It is generally a disease of later life, more often affecting 6% to 8% of adults over 65 years of age. It has a major impact on health care costs and the nation overall, with costs ranging to more than $100 billion per year. Immeasurable is the impact and the emotional and physical toll it has on patients, their families, and the community at large.[1]

The general public misperception about dementia is that a majority of the individuals are diagnosed and cared for in acute and long-term care facility settings; this assumption is far from the truth. A majority of patients with dementia are living at home with caregivers who are themselves over 50 years of age, have little to no medical training, and have few financial resources to support the care needed. When medical issues arise, health care access is difficult at best. Considering the limited access to health care the elderly have overall in society and taking into account the overall shortage of geriatricians, neurologists, and psychiatrists trained in these specialties, primary care providers are usually on the front lines in the diagnosis and care of these patients.

Gwinnett Health Systems, 1000 Medical Center Boulevard, Lawrenceville, GA 30046, USA
E-mail address: mdarrow@gwinnettmedicalcenter.org

Prim Care Clin Office Pract 42 (2015) 195–204
http://dx.doi.org/10.1016/j.pop.2015.01.008
0095-4543/15/$ – see front matter © 2015 Elsevier Inc. All rights reserved.

This article suggests an effective and economical approach to the primary care work-up of patients with dementia, including the diagnosis and treatment modalities available to primary care providers.[2]

## DEFINITIONS AND THE TYPES OF DEMENTIA

Dementia is generally defined as a significant deterioration in 2 or more areas of cognitive function that results in an overall functional decline of an individual. The following is a list of the more commonly found and agreed-on syndromes.

### Mild Cognitive Impairment

There has recently been interest in mild cognitive impairment as a possible prodromal marker for dementia. Patients with mild cognitive impairment are individuals who have sustained identifiable cognitive deficiencies but are still quite functional. It has been observed that approximately 10% of these patients per year "go onto" to some identifiable form of dementia compared with a 1% to 2% conversion rate in the population over age 85 with no cognitive impairment. Although this diagnosis has over time been confused with normal physiologic aging and other entities, the basic criteria seem clear and include sustained cognitive complaints that can be documented by cognitive testing in the presence of generally preserved activities of daily living (ADLs).

### Alzheimer Disease

Alzheimer disease (AD) is the most common cause of dementia. Although a conclusive diagnosis is made by pathologic identification of senile plaques and neurofibrillary tangles, accepted clinical criteria are now available to assist in the diagnosis. Traditionally, AD is characterized by gradual-onset memory, language, and visual spatial impairments and gradual progression of 8 to 10 years, with motor skills remaining intact until very late in the progression of the disease.

### Vascular Dementia

Vascular dementia (VD) is seen as sudden or stepwise in progression; it is often associated with vascular changes to the brain. It accounts for 15% to 20% of the dementias observed. The affected cognitive functions depend on the location of the neurologic injury as do the affected motor skills. This injury is often associated with clinically visible neurologic changes. Progression, like onset, is often gradual or stepwise with continued vascular insult.

### Lewy Body Dementia

Lewy body dementia (LBD) may overlap with the dementia associated with Parkinson disease and AD and, therefore, has been until recent years difficult to understand. Its onset is gradual; there are deficits in memory, visual spatial relationships, and hallucinations. Generally, there is fluctuation of all of these symptoms over time. The motor findings are those commonly seen in parkinsonism, in particular the pill-rolling tremor and muscular rigidity. When these physical signs develop with or after the onset of the dementia, LBD is to be considered.

### Frontotemporal Dementia

Frontotemporal dementia (FTD) is often seen at a younger age than the other dementia syndromes. Patients with FTD have gradual onset of behavioral and language symptoms. Memory may be affected but often to a much lesser degree than those individuals with AD. Behavioral changes are mostly striking and include disinhibition, impulsivity, and increased and often pressured speech. Patients with AD may have "frontal symptoms," but memory issues in AD present early on and the behavioral problems are much later in onset, where the opposite is true for FTD. Pick disease is a form of FTD associated with balloon-like inclusions in brain cells at autopsy. Neuronal intermediate filament inclusion disorder (NIFID) is another subclass of FTD. The mean age of onset of NIFID is approximately 40 years.

Less common causes of dementia, such as those associated with Parkinson disease, Creutzfeldt-Jakob disease, Huntington chorea, hippocampal sclerosis, and other neurodegenerative diseases and with metabolic and genetic deficiencies, are not discussed in this article and have been associated with laboratory, pathologic, and/or clinical signs identifying their presentation. Reversible causes of dementia make up less than 2% of cases and are also often identified during a work-up.[3,4]

## DIAGNOSIS AND WORK-UP

The dementia work-up has gone through much scrutiny and modification over time such that in general, at this time, it is recommended that this evaluation occurs over at least 2 office visits and should involve gathering as much information and input as possible for diagnosis and treatment from as many sources and points of view as are available. The first step in the work-up is to determine whether a true dementia exists. It is common for an individual to present with "benign forgetfulness" or occasional memory complaints commonly seen with advancing age. These symptoms are not sustained and are not associated with a decline in function. They are often noticed when an individual's attention is diverted, split among multiple tasks, or compromised in some fashion. Commonly, the complaint is inability to remember names or the location of certain objects and items. Although this may occur with some regularity in a given individual, it is not a precursor to dementia or an early presentation of dementia.[5]

It is generally accepted that the dementia syndromes are classified by their risk factors, characteristic findings, and progressive clinical degenerative changes. The clinical assessment of dementia involves the gathering of as much information as possible from patients, loved ones, friends, and others (**Table 1**). With all types of dementia, cognitive impairment is progressive, is persistent, and has a profound effect on patient ADLs and instrumental ADLs (IADLs), such that even casual observations may be helpful and informative in an evaluation. Most dementias can be diagnosed by general medical and psychiatric evaluations performed by an alert primary care physician.

**Table 1**
**Differential diagnosis and summary**

| Syndrome | Onset | Cognitive Symptoms | Motor Symptoms | Progression |
|----------|-------|--------------------|----------------|-------------|
| AD | Gradual | Memory, visuospatial | Apraxia very late | 8–10 y |
| VD | Stepwise | Location specific | Correlates to ischemia | Stepwise with ischemia |
| LBD | Gradual | Memory, hallucinations | Parkinson like | 6–8 y |
| FTD | Gradual, younger patients | Disinhibition | Few | 6–8 y |

*Adapted from* Pascala JT. Geriatrics Review Syllabus (GRS7). American Geriatric Society; 2010.

Behavioral disturbances often precede the onset of most dementias. **Box 1** lists the most common early subjective complaints presented by either patients or families.[6]

## Complete History and Functional Tests

The use of office-based assessment tools is essential in the evaluation. In addition to patients themselves, a close and reliable informant can be an excellent source of information on these patients, in particular their current condition, medical condition, medication history, patterns of substance abuse, living arrangements, and ADLs and IADLs. Timing of onset and the nature of symptoms are critical and help differentiate clinical syndromes. Besides a thorough history, other important common tools are functional activity assessment tools. Cognition should be assessed with cognitive function tests, such as the Mini-Mental State Examination, the Montreal Cognitive Assessment, and the Saint Louis University Mental Status Examination. The presence of depression should also be screened for using depression scales, screening tools, and assessment. Families' and friends' observations can and should be used when screening with these instruments or by direct questioning.[7]

## Physical Examination

The physical examination should be extensive enough to include those areas that may demonstrate deficiencies indicating physical, neurologic, or other systemic symptoms and characteristics that may point to concurrent causative processes.

## Laboratories as Part of the Standard Work-up

Unless guided by history and physical examination findings, the laboratory studies listed in **Box 2** are recommended.

The emerging field of biomarkers and their use in the early detection of AD are discussed briefly. Increasing knowledge is being gained about proteins and peptide groups that seem consistently present in varied amounts in patients with AD. Although it is probable that these markers will, in the future, be useful in the early detection and treatment of dementia, at this time and at the current level of understanding and ability to intervene, they seem to have little utility in the primary care setting in the diagnosis and work-up of dementia.[5]

## Imaging

A CT of the head without contrast is generally adequate in a routine dementia work-up to exclude issues commonly part of the differential diagnosis of dementia, such as an intracranial bleed, normal pressure hydrocephalus, and so forth. It is agreed, however, that more extensive imaging studies, such as MRI and magnetic

---

**Box 1**
**Common complaints preceding dementia**

1. Behavioral changes
2. Missed deadlines at work or home
3. Other work-related problems
4. Difficulty in managing complex tasks, such as finances
5. The abandonment of hobbies or other interests

> **Box 2**
> **Recommended laboratory studies**
>
> - Complete blood cell count
> - Urine analysis
> - Serum chemistries
> - Liver function tests
> - Vitamin $B_{12}$ and folate levels
> - Thyroid-stimulating hormone

resonance angiography, may be useful in patients with the following characteristics or findings:

- Dementia onset less than 65 years of age
- Sudden or rapid progression of symptoms
- Presentation with a focal neurologic deficit
- A clinical picture consistent with normal pressure hydrocephalus
- Experiencing a recent full or head trauma

More specific or functional imaging, such as PET scanning, is recommended only if a diagnosis remains uncertain and, at that point, specialty consultation is likely needed.[8]

## TREATMENT AND MANAGEMENT

The treatment and management of dementia should have the primary goal of maintaining the highest quality of life possible for patients and those in the support system around them. Providers should ensure that there is maximization of patient functional performance by improving and or stabilizing cognition, mood, and behavior. Only mild cognitive improvement is usually achieved and that it is transient at best. Providers must, therefore, set realistic, reasonable, and well-informed expectations of patients, family members, and support systems. The initial treatment strategy should always be a nonpharmacologic one that takes full advantage of available multidisciplinary resources and tools. Because all dementias are progressive, resulting in eventual cognitive decline with loss of function, the use of pharmacologic interventions should be limited to assisting in decreasing the risk of physical violence, extreme patient distress, and depression, with a particular goal of preserving a specific level of function. Once this level of functioning is lost, there should be no hesitation in discontinuing the pharmacologic interventions because their prolonged usage can be detrimental over time. Lastly, because dementia and functional loss progress, any sudden acute change may likely represent undiagnosed medical problems, pain, depression, anxiety, sleeplessness, or delirium, to name a few of the common causes, and should not lead to more long-term interventions until the urgent issue is identified and resolved.[9]

### Nonpharmacologic Treatment

The nonpharmacologic treatment approach should be the first intervention considered and explored. There are many approaches:

### Cognitive rehabilitation

New learning skills are lost early on in most of the dementia syndromes, rendering techniques, such as reality orientation, memory training, and other types of cognitive rehabilitation, essentially ineffective and often leading to increased anxiety on the part of everyone involved.[2]

### Supportive therapy

Reminiscence therapy and social activities, such as dancing, singing, and other recreational activities are effective in redirecting anxiety and depression and in assisting resolving behavioral symptoms. Support groups may be useful early in the course of dementia particularly for behavioral problems and mood swings experienced by patients and those in their support system. Physical therapy, more specifically physical activity and exercise, should be encouraged because there is some evidence showing these activities have an effect on motivation, behaviors, and cognition. Manipulative therapy may be useful in some cases especially where pain, stiffness, and other musculoskeletal problems may be causing discomfort or anxiety.[10]

### Regular appointments and family and caregiver support

Support and ongoing education are essential for all of those affected by dementia. Regularly scheduled visits every 3 to 6 months to address ongoing comorbidities; behavioral, functional, and emotional issues; safety instruction; and attention to environmental changes and issues are essential. If patients are on a medication, evaluation as to its effectiveness and potential side effect and the possibility of drug-free periods should be considered.

### Caregiver well-being and education

Addressing a caregiver's well-being and concerns at each visit should not be forgotten. Community resources for support and management can allow families and loved ones a chance to cope more efficiently. Inquiries into financial management, health care proxy availability, and advanced care directives must be performed and addressed. Discussions about long-term care and other future needs should occur early on in the course of treatment to allow an informed thought process, financial planning, and alignment of the proper support system, goals of treatment, and therapy.[11]

### Environmental preparation and safety

Patients with dementia are influenced greatly by their environment. At least 1 home visit may be extremely useful to providers in assessing patient surroundings. The following steps are generally recommended in the treatment course[10]:

- Prevention of overstimulation with a goal of moderate stimulation
- Use of familiar surroundings, such as pictures and old furniture
- The introduction of as much routine into daily activities as possible
- The use of visual and other familiar cues, such as stop signs on outside doors and pictures on the outside of rooms, for identification can have a great impact on reducing anxiety.
- Attention to safety, such as locking dangerous areas and use of nametags and pass codes on a unit, is needed.
- The evaluation of the ability of patients to drive and operate a motor vehicle in the outpatient setting is often difficult at best for providers, patients, and loved ones but is an important safety intervention.

### Additional resources

Community support for dementia patients, neighbors, and friends is often key and critical. This support can be the informal support of neighborhoods, family service agencies, adult day care centers and networks, church support groups, and other social groups. The availability of specialized services, such as adult day care, respite care, and home health agencies, can provide important nursing support. Organizations, such as the Alzheimer's Association, and other outreach services offered by local agencies and councils of aging may also be available. Meals on Wheels and similar food services for homebound individuals are often available. Meal and other domestic support may also be available from local senior citizen centers, church and community groups, and some local health care institutions. Transportation is commonly offered with some of these services as well. Providers should make themselves familiar with all of the potentially available resources to assist in the support of these patients.[11]

## Pharmacologic Treatment

When prescribing medications to patients with dementia, providers must keep in mind the following principles:

- Virtually all groups of medications have been known to lead to issues in the elderly, dementia aside.
- Wide variation and response to medications are often the rule.
- When introducing a drug, start at a low dose and increase it slowly over time.
- Assessment of the continued use of any medication with cognitive and functional goals is essential.
- Nonpharmacologic intervention, such as distraction, misdirection, and organized activities, can be effective and may be superior to medication in many acute situations.

Issues commonly leading to the use of medications in patients with dementia are cognitive function stabilization and enhancement, depression, anxiety, and psychiatric issues. There has been much attention given over the years to the side effects of medications and the morbidity and mortality of the elderly. The Beers list is the most commonly used reference in this area. It contains the current understanding, recommendations, and potential issues of medications in all of the major categories used in the care of elderly patients.[12]

### Cognitive enhancement medications

The most commonly prescribed medications for cognitive enhancement are the cholinesterase inhibitors (CIs) (**Table 2**). These medications are useful in the stabilization of cognitive function but have demonstrated only a moderate delay in cognitive decline. The same can be said for their effect on behavioral problems and function. The recommendation for their use is essentially limited to patients with AD, although they may have some utility in the treatment of hallucinations associated with LBD. The use of CIs in patients with VD and FTD is not recommended. Reassessment of patients for continued drug effectiveness and potential side effects is recommended every 3 to 6 months.

Table 2
**Cholinesterase inhibitors prescribed for cognitive enhancement**

| Drug | Initial Dose | Titration |
|------|-------------|-----------|
| Donepezil | 5 mg qd for 4–6 wk | Increase to maximum of 10 mg qd |
| Rivastigmine | 1.5 mg bid, double as indicated | Maximum dose of 6 mg bid |
| Galantamine | 4 mg bid for 4 wk | Maximum of 12 mg q 12 h |
| Memantine | 5 mg qd for 1 wk | Increase to bid dosing and maximum of 10 mg bid |

Other cognitive-enhancing preparations, such as antioxidants, gingko balboa, and vitamin E, seem to consistently cause unusual side effects and studies have not demonstrated significant benefit to improving cognition; they are not recommended.[12]

### Antidepressants

Antidepressant medications should be considered in patients with AD and depressive symptoms. The symptoms can include depressed mood, loss of appetite, fatigue, sleeplessness, irritability, and agitation. Selective serotonin reuptake inhibitor (SSRI) medications should be considered. Sertraline and citalopram have demonstrated some efficacy in this regard. Additionally, SSRIs may be helpful in patients with FTD and compulsive or disinhibited behaviors.

### Medications for behavioral syndromes

Manic-like symptoms may from time to time be present in dementia patients. These episodes are similar to those experienced by bipolar patients and may respond to the common therapies used to treat bipolar disorder. Specific goals for therapy and a short treatment course should be considered. Divalproex sodium, carbamazepine, lamotrigine, and lithium also may be considered.

### Sedative and psychoactive medications

Sedative and psychoactive medications probably are the most misunderstood yet most commonly used class in the care of patients with dementia. The medications listed in **Table 3** may be used on a time-limited basis for specific issues, such as the presence of delusions, hallucinations, paranoia, and, occasionally, the irritability associated with these disorders. They are for those situations that potentially lead to harm of patients and their caregivers. Careful consideration of the causes of a behavior as well as nonpharmacologic treatment approaches must be done before their use given their anticholinergic properties and linkage to falls, increased mortality, and neurologic side effects. Use of the lowest effective dose possible is the best approach. Primary sleep disturbances that are not responsive to behavioral interventions also may be treated with medications on a time-limited basis.

### When to Refer

The types and availability of specialty referral resources available to primary care physicians in the care of dementia patients should also be common knowledge for the successful treatment of patients with dementia. A referral to a specialist for specialty consultative services is important and, in some situations, extremely important. Some general recommendations as to when referral may be helpful are listed in **Box 3**.[13–15]

| Table 3 Sedative and psychoactive medications | | |
|---|---|---|
| **Drug** | **Starting Dose** | **Indication** |
| Risperdone | 5 mg | AD with psychosis for at least 1 mo |
| Olanzapine | 2.5 mg | AD with psychosis for at least 1 mo |
| Quetiapine | 25 mg | AD with psychosis for at least 1 mo |
| Aripiprazole | 5 mg | AD with psychosis for at least 1 mo |
| Trazodone | 25 mg | Sleep disturbances not responsive to behavioral management |
| Mirtazapine | 7.5 mg | Sleep disturbances not responsive to behavioral management |
| Zolpidem | 5 mg | Sleep disturbances not responsive to behavioral management |
| Zaleplon | 5 mg | Sleep disturbances not responsive to behavioral management |

> **Box 3**
> **Recommendations for when to refer patients**
>
> 1. Unusual or atypical presentation
> 2. Onset of dementia before age 60
> 3. Overwhelming psychological or behavioral issues that are difficult to manage
> 4. Depression with violence or suicidal behaviors

### Specialists

Neurologists are commonly engaged in the care of patients with overwhelming parkinsonian features, focal neurologic signs and symptoms, or unusually rapid progression of their disease process.

Neuropsychological consultation can help clarify diagnostically complex cases, and clinical psychologists can provide support to patients but, most importantly, the caregivers.

Social workers are important in explaining, contacting, and engaging community as well as engaging patients and families in discussions of financial support and other legal matters.

Nurse case management and intervention can guide behavior management, feeding, and other critical issues.

Clinical pharmacologists, when available, help minimize adverse drug events, assist caregivers' administration of medications, and assist providers with the initiation and/or withdrawal of medications.

Legal experts and attorneys should assist in the construction of wills, conservatorships, trusts, health care power of attorney, estate planning, and other legal matters as required.

### SUMMARY

The care of patients with dementia is a common need in the primary setting and a unique opportunity for providers to evaluate and treat patients and their families and loved ones while utilizing simple and common approaches using available community resources. This approach also presents individuals with a focused, 1-provider, patient-centered, and tailored treatment plan. The diagnostic tools used are common, simple, and readily available. The treatments are multiple and multidisciplinary. As the population ages, this approach will become more popular and essential in the care of dementia patients and their families in a community setting.

### REFERENCES

1. Brayne C, Fox C, Boustani M. Dementia screening in primary care, is it time? JAMA 2007;298(20):2409–11.
2. Morris JC. Dementia update 2005. Alzheimer Dis Assoc Disord 2005;19(2): 110–7.
3. Knopman DS, Dekosky ST, Cummings JL, et al. Practice parameter: diagnosis of dementia (an evidence based review). Report of the Quality of Standards Sub-Committee of the American Academy of Neurology. Neurology 2001;56:1143–53.
4. Boustani M, Peterson B, Hanson L, et al. Screening for Dementia. Systematic evidence review. Available at: http://www.ahrq.gov/clinic/uspstfix.htm. Accessed October 10, 2007.

5. Corner L, Bond J. Being at risk of dementia: fears and anxieties of older adults. J Aging Stud 2004;18(2):143–55.
6. Holsinger R, Deveau J, Boustani M, et al. Does this patient have dementia? JAMA 2007;297(21):2391–404.
7. Markwick A, Zamboni G, de Jager CA. Profiles of cognitive Assessment (MoCA) in a research cohort with normal Mini-mental State Examination (MMSE) scores. J Clin Exp Neuropsychol 2012;34(7):750–7.
8. Galasko D. The diagnostic evaluation of a patient with dementia. Continuum 2013;19(2 Dementia):397–410.
9. Cooper C, Mukadam N, Katona C, et al. Systemic review of the effectiveness of pharmacologic interventions to improve quality of life and well-being in people with dementia. Am J Geriatr Psychiatry 2013;21(2):173–83.
10. Lawrence V, Fossey J, Ballard C, et al. Improving quality of life for people with dementia in care home: making psychological interventions work. Br J Psychiatry 2012;201:344–51.
11. Yaffe K, Hoang T. Non-pharmacologic treatment and prevention strategies for dementia. Continuum 2013;19(2 Dementia):372–81.
12. The American Geriatrics Society 2012 Beers Criteria Update Expert Panel. American Geriatrics Society Updated Beers Criteria for potentially inappropriate medication use in older adults. J Am Geriatr Soc 2012;60(4):616–31.
13. Agosta F, Caso F, Filippi M. Dementia and neuroimaging. J Neurol 2013;260(2):685–91.
14. Manthorpe J, Samsi K, Campbell S, et al. From forgetfulness to dementia: clinical and commissioning implications of diagnostic experiences. Br J Clin Pract 2013;63(606):e69–75.
15. Simmons BB, Hartmann B, DeJoseph D. Evaluation of suspected dementia. Am Fam Physician 2011;84(8):895–902.

# Approach to the Patient with Parkinson Disease

Kevin E. Johnson, MD

## KEYWORDS

- Parkinson disease • Diagnosis • Treatment • Motor symptoms
- Nonmotor symptoms

## KEY POINTS

- Progressive neurodegenerative disease is characterized pathologically by changes in the mesencephalic substantia nigra and physiologically by development of cardinal motor symptoms of resting tremor, bradykinesia, and rigidity, and eventually postural instability.
- All current treatment is based on symptom management, as no effective cure or disease modification is currently available.
- Appropriate diagnosis and periodic reassessment are critical to assure appropriate therapy and avoid mistreatment and delay in addressing other conditions with overlapping symptoms.
- Supporting the patient and caregiver holistically is important, as significant comorbid conditions related to the disease can impact quality of life and relationships; addressing psychological and support needs along with physical symptoms is critical to providing effective care.

First Described in 1817 by James Parkinson as a neurologic disorder primarily affecting musculoskeletal function and preserving senses and intellect, Parkinson disease (PD) is currently understood as a progressive neurodegenerative disease with motor, nonmotor, and behavioral findings. Significant advances in imaging technology have allowed the characterization of the underlying pathologic changes to the mesencephalic substantia nigra, and development of alpha-synuclein containing Lewy bodies in the remaining dopaminergic neurons. Although certain imaging techniques currently allow for detection in some patients as much as 20 years prior to the onset of motor symptoms, these advances have yet to produce a meaningful treatment to halt the progression of the disease or reverse its course. Current treatments are directed at optimizing symptomatic management.[1,2]

Disclosures: The author has nothing to disclose.
Family Medicine Residency, Gwinnett Medical Center, 665 Duluth Hwy, Suite 501, Lawrenceville, GA 30046, USA
E-mail address: kejohnson@gwinnettmedicalcenter.org

Prim Care Clin Office Pract 42 (2015) 205–215
http://dx.doi.org/10.1016/j.pop.2015.01.005

The incidence of PD varies with age, commonly cited as approximately 1% by the sixth decade of life, and approaching 4% by the end of the eighth decade of life. Although the disease may occur as early as the teenage years, with disease occurring before the second decade of life labeled as juvenile-onset and between the second and fourth decades as young-onset, the average age at diagnosis is 70.5 years.[3] White, non-Hispanic persons living in the Midwest and northeastern United States are disproportionately represented in epidemiologic studies by review of claims data.[4]

## CAUSATIVE AND PREDICTIVE FACTORS

Research into genetic factors and identification of environmental risk factors have yet to provide a definitive predictive model for PD. A positive family history is a risk factor for PD, with first-degree relatives of PD patients 2.3 times more likely to develop PD.[5] Genetic studies continue to identify numerous heritable forms of the disease, designated with PARK1, PARK2, and similar designations, with various autosomal-dominant, x-linked, and autosomal-recessive families. Despite these advances, most cases at this writing remain sporadic in nature.[6] Observational and case–control studies and meta-analysis of environmental risk factors support correlation with exposures to pesticides and herbicides, along with exposure to well water, living on a farm, and exposure to farm animals.[7,8] Protective exposures have also been studied, including smoking and coffee drinking.[9] Despite the noted risk reduction of smoking for PD, other health risks still preclude recommending smoking as a preventative measure.

## DIAGNOSTIC GOLD STANDARD STILL ELUSIVE

Because no definitive laboratory and radiological test with gold standard level specificity for PD currently exists, history and physical examination remain the cornerstones of diagnosis. Classic cardinal motor symptoms of resting tremor, bradykinesia, and rigidity, and eventually postural instability, form the basis for the initial diagnosis of idiopathic PD (**Box 1**). Early disease can be easily misdiagnosed because of the relative vagueness of symptoms and mistaking early signs for normal aging processes.[10] Understanding the complex interaction of motor, cognitive, behavioral/neuropsychiatric, and autonomic dysfunction, as well as significant overlap with other neurodegenerative processes associated with tremor, makes a high index of suspicion and a broad differential diagnosis important in the clinical evaluation.

Most current practice guidelines for PD suggest referral to a physician with expertise in movement disorders should be considered for physicians who are unsure or lack experience in the initial diagnosis of PD. Because treatment may mask the clinical diagnostic features and further delay definitive diagnosis, consideration should be given to referral before initiation of treatment. Despite the lack of definitive outcome-based studies or cost-benefit analyses that demonstrate definite benefit of this approach, the significant psychological stress of the diagnosis of a chronic progressive neurologic disease with such profound impacts makes judgment in favor of early referral warranted, especially in cases where the diagnosis is unclear, in the younger patient, or rapid or unusual progression of symptoms. Periodic reassessment of the diagnosis should also be done for all patients to evaluate for possible misdiagnosis.[11] **Table 1** provides a partial list of diseases often misdiagnosed as PD.[1,12–14]

The natural course of idiopathic PD is a progressive decline in motor and cognitive function, with a contaminant rise in morbidity and mortality related to both. Changes in cognition are most closely related to patient age at diagnosis, and duration of disease and early or rapid progression of dementia may suggest an alternative diagnosis. One large review of mortality studies showed an average shortening of life expectancy ranging from 3 years in patients over 65, to 11 years of lost life expectancy for those diagnosed before the age of 40.[15]

## MANAGEMENT

In rare instances, PD can be rapidly progressive. The usual course is more gradual, with patients who can survive decades with slow but eventually significant change in disease severity and symptomatology. Patients benefit from physicians who understand the progression and symptoms of early and progressive PD; have a knowledge of current therapies for PD, especially the effects of medications, along with their adverse effects; and have an awareness of medications that can interact with PD treatments and cause significant morbidity and even mortality.

Although memorization of a list of drugs with potential interactions with PD and treatments for it can be a useful safety check, the main classes of medications that are generally contraindicated for PD fall into 3 main classes: antipsychotics, antidepressants, and antiemetics (especially anticholinergic ones). It is important that all physicians prescribing for PD patients consider the risk of any new medication. Integrated drug–drug and drug–disease interaction checking is one of the meaningful use requirements for Centers for Medicare Services outpatient electronic health record incentive, and promises the potential to be an important safety step for prescribing.[16] Although proof that drug–drug interaction is a significant source of harm exists in the literature, studies demonstrating improved outcomes clinically from outpatient use of electronic interaction checking are not robust in their current evidence.

Initial treatment of PD for most newly diagnosed mild-to-moderate cases of PD involves a coordinated effort to educate the patient and caregivers about support services, disease processes, and exercise for general health and conditioning. Evidence also suggests that the gains from exercise may be lost if activity is not maintained on a regular basis.[17,18] Although some studies have suggested that early physical therapy for PD, a systematic review demonstrated short-term gains in gait and walking measures, but was inconclusive for demonstrated benefit in fall reduction or patient-reported quality of life.[19,20]

When to initiate treatment with medication is a somewhat controversial, as most current disease management guideline recommendations suggest waiting until the disease progresses to a point that the patient is functionally impaired. Given the lack of conclusively proven neuroprotective effect of any currently available medication, despite several early promising trials, there is no currently accepted preventive medication available for PD. The PD LIFE audit , a multicentre longitudinal observational study of changes in self reported health status in people with Parkinson's disease left untreated at diagnosis, did demonstrate a favorable quality of life outcome at 18 months for patients treated with dopaminergic medications over an untreated cohort.[19]

## TREATMENT OF MOTOR SYMPTOMS OF PARKINSON DISEASE

Choice of an initial agent for treatment of PD depends on risk and benefit evaluations, which much be considered individually and discussed with the patient and/or caregiver. The goal of improving motor function and decreasing debility generally attributed to dopamine deficiency must also be compared with the risk of motor complications, exacerbation of neuropsychiatric symptoms, and dementia, in addition to unique adverse effects of certain classes and individual medications. Preference for certain agents and classes of medications will be discussed.

Levodopa is a precursor drug to dopamine that is converted both peripherally and centrally and is given in combination with carbidopa, which prevents levodopa's

**Box1**
**Clinical features in Parkinson disease**

Motor:

- Tremor[a]
- Bradykinesia[a]
- Rigidity[a]
- Gait disturbances[a]
- Balance problems
- Stooped posture
- Micrographia[b]
- Dystonia
- Myoclonus
- Difficulty turning in bed

Craniofacial:

- Hypomimia (Masked facies, reduced expression)
- Dysphagia (difficulty with swallowing)
- Speech impairments
- Sialorrhea (drooling)[b]
- Rhinorrhea
- Eyelid opening apraxia
- Gaze abnormalities

Sensation:

- Anosmia (loss of smell)[b]
- Blurred vision
- Pain
- Parathesias

Neuropsychiatric:

- Fatigue[b]
- Cognitive dysfunction/dementia
- Psychosis
- Hallucinations
- Depression
- Anxiety
- Apathy
- Sleep disturbance

Autonomic dysfunction:

- Constipation[b]
- Urinary urgency
- Nocturia
- Sexual dysfunction

Other:

- Seborrheic dermatitis

[a] Cardinal features.
[b] May occur decades before Dx.

peripheral conversion, reducing dose-limiting adverse effects such and nausea and vomiting. The combination is available in several dosages, in both long-acting and immediate-release formulations, and the short-acting formulation requires 3 times daily dosage for effect. Because of its low cost and high initial efficacy, it remains among the most popular choice for initiation of monotherapy, especially in the older patient population. Its primary drawback is the gradual increase in motor fluctuations, both abrupt and gradual, along with random on-off effects that tend to occur initially after 4 to 5 years of treatment. Dyskinesias can also occur with levodopa, and are usually related to peak dose effects. In later stage disease, the dopaminergic effects can also manifest as worsening of neuropsychiatric symptoms, including psychosis and hallucinations, which may eventually require reduction or discontinuation. Because of these issues, consideration of other initial agents is important in younger PD patients, given the probable longevity of their disease.[14]

Nonergot dopamine agonists (DAs) pramipexole, and ropinirole can be used in early PD or as add on therapy in later disease. These medications are longer-acting in duration and are less likely to cause wearing-off or dyskinesia untoward effects; however,

**Table 1**
**Diseases often misdiagnosed as Parkinson disease**

| Condition | Features That Favor Condition Over Idiopathic PD |
|---|---|
| Essential tremor | Family history, faster frequency of tremor, normal facial expression, responds to alcohol, worsens with intent |
| Drug-induced parkinsonism | History of causative drug use (antipsychotics, antiemetics) Withdrawal of drug can confirm Dx. |
| Multisystem degenerations (parkinsonism-plus) Examples: <br> • Progressive supernuclear palsy <br> • Multiple system atrophy | Cerebellar signs, supranuclear gaze palsy, dystonia |
| Vascular parkinsonism | Stepwise progression, localizing neurologic findings on exam, lacunar infarcts on computed tomography/MRI |
| Inherited neurodegenerative Parkinsonism Examples: <br> • Wilson disease <br> • Huntington disease | Positive Family history, abnormal LFTs, Kayser–Fleischer rings, wing-flapping tremor, seziures, chorea |
| Pugilistic encephalopathy | History of repeated head trauma (classically boxing) |
| Lewy body dementia | Onset of dementia/psychiatric symptoms before onset of motor symptoms |

*Data from* Refs.[1,12–14]

peripheral effects of dopamine such as nausea, hypotension, edema, and somnolence, along with possible neuropsychiatric adverse effects, including impulse control disorders such as hypersexuality and compulsive gambling must be discussed with patients at length before starting these medications. Although levodopa has been proven more efficacious for motor symptoms in multiple trials, individuals with mild motor symptoms who favor less pill burden, and especially younger patients who are more likely to develop eventual side effects from levodopa due to longer term use may benefit from a trial of these medications initially.[21] Older ergot DA medications such as bromocriptine have significant risk of adverse effects including retroperitoneal and pulmonary fibrosis with long-term use. DA medications also increase treatment costs over levodopa.

Monoamine oxidase B (MAO-B) inhibitors selegiline, and rasagiline are also considered effective in montherapy for PD. In the brain, dopamine is broken down by MAO-B, and inhibition of this breakdown increases dopamine's availability. Although generally less effective than levodopa, most clinicians also feel that MAO-B inhibitors are clinically inferior to DAs, although reviews of trial data do not definitively show superiority of the DAs. MAO-B inhibitors can also be used as add-on therapy with levodopa to treat motor complications. A large prospective trial of rasagiline with a delayed start design was recently completed showing ambiguous results with regards to neuroprotective effects, although a 24-month trial is currently underway that may provide more insight to the potential of this pathway for early intervention. Consideration must also be given to the cost and potential adverse effects of the medications, including risk of withdrawal syndrome and tyramine-containing foods.[22]

Anticholinergic medications, including benztropine and trihexaphenidyl, represent older-generation PD treatments that are not generally considered first-line but occasionally are used for resistant cases of tremor and in younger patients who can tolerate the adverse effects of dry eyes and mouth, urinary retention, and constipation. They are generally contraindicated in older patients because of worsening of cognitive function along with other effects.[23]

Catechol-O-methyl transferase (COMT) inhibitors entacapone and tolcapone are used to reduce the metabolism of levodopa to maintain "on" time, and entacapone also exists in a combination with levodopa/carbidopa to reduce total pill burden and therefore compliance. Severe diarrhea is the most common adverse effect and may prevent use of these medications in some individuals; tolcapone can also induce fatal hepatotoxicity and is contraindicated in individuals with pre-existing liver disease and requires monitoring of transaminanses at regular intervals and prompt discontinuation if abnormal changes in hepatic function tests are noted.[2,23]

Amantadine is an NMDA glutamate receptor blocker with a proposed ability to cause presynaptic release of dopamine. Initially approved for influenza treatment, it has been used for add-on therapy for both anticholinergics and levodopa with evidence of benefit, although the gains have been of relatively modest duration in most individuals. Adverse effects can include the typical anticholinergic constellation, along with livedo reticularis, anorexia, and insomnia.[11]

## SURGICAL TREATMENT OPTIONS

Patients who have continued to progress to the point of significant disability or have significant adverse effects from optimal medical therapy but are young and healthy enough may be candidates for surgical deep brain stimulation (DBS). Although the risk of adverse events is significant, approaching 50% in some randomized controlled trials, results can provide a significant improvement in function, reduced medication requirements, and provide several more years of function for a select group of patients.[11,24]

## NONMOTOR TREATMENT CONSIDERATIONS

Primary care physicians should pay special attention to subtle signs of changes in mood and affect in PD patients, as the incidence of neuropsychiatric symptoms increases with the duration of disease, and can often be dismissed or denied by the patient and caregiver. Masked facies can also pose a potential challenge, as visual clues physicians are trained to use to help recognize anxiety, depression and other mood disorders are often lost or severely attenuated.

Caregiver fatigue and burnout can also pose a substantial risk for patient caregiver dyads, especially if the caregiver is an older spouse also dealing with health issues. Continual education is important, along with support services referrals.

## DEMENTIA

PD dementia (PDD) is a common late manifestation of PD, and given the increased life expectancy seen with improved optimization of motor symptom management and overall care, the incidence is reported as reaching cumulative levels of up to 80%. PDD shares many features with Lewy body dementia (LBD), including hallucinations that may predate the cognitive decline and impulsivity that can manifest as hypersexuality or compulsive gambling can also occur. Sleep is additionally often disrupted. Careful evaluation of the patient should be done to preclude other causes of dementia.

The cholinesterase inhibitors rivastigmine and donepezil have both been shown to have beneficial effects on cognition in PDD; side effects of nausea, urinary retention, and worsening of tremor may significantly limit their clinical usefulness.[25] Memetidine has been found to have limited effectiveness in LBD, but no significant effect when used in PDD.[26–28] Consideration should also be given to reduction in anticholinergic drug use for motor symptoms in an effort to delay worsening of cognitive decline.[25]

## PSYCHOSIS

Hallucinations, as noted previously, are relatively common in PD, and may predate cognitive decline. Withdrawal of medications, which may be exacerbating hallucinations, and careful evaluation for sources of metabolic disturbance and infection are warranted as well. Clozapine has been documented in several large trials, although monitoring of cardiac and hematological function is mandatory given significant risks. Providers and pharmacies must enroll in a restricted distribution program. Quetiapine has also been studied with conflicting data between studies, but clinically it offers the best potential adverse effect profile. Other newer atypical antipsychotics all produce significant motor worsening and are not recommended. Rivastigmine and donepezil have also shown some benefit for hallucinations.[25] Low-dose intravenous benzodiazepines such as lorazepam have been used in emergent situations. Haloperidol, olanzapine, and risperidone should all be avoided, as severe rigidity can be induced.[1]

## DEPRESSION

Depression related to PD is a frequent comorbidity and can be a challenging problem. Because of the significant symptom overlap, diagnosis can be more difficult. Reduced facial expression can limit sensitivity of observation for flattened affect; progression of motor symptoms can be confused for loss of energy, tremor for psychomotor agitation, or medication effects for motor slowing. A high index of suspicion and a screening tool are recommended due to prevalence and high morbidity and mortality associated with untreated depression.

Selective serotonin reuptake inhibitors have mixed evidence as to their effectiveness, although due to their favorable adverse effect profile they have been used clinically and are worth therapeutic trial before considering older tricyclic antidepressants (TCAs). TCAs, especially nortriptyline and desipramine, have limited studies which demonstrate some efficacy, and the dopamine agonist pramipexole has also been shown to have antidepressant effects in PD that are not just related to its motor effects. Careful monitoring for suicidal and homicidal ideations and prompt specialty consultation should be considered.

## SLEEP

Sleep disorders in PD can take a variety of forms. Fatigue is one of the most common complaints in PD, and a careful history can help elucidate possible causes and treatments. Common issues seen include daytime somnolence, which can vary from mild to hazardous sleep attacks, and occurs in more than half of all PD affected individuals. This can be related to disease-related or treatment-related issues and can be linked to nighttime sleep disturbances in many PD patients. Modafinil has been studied and shown mixed data for effectiveness in isolated daytime somnolence and can be considered for therapy.[29] Methylphenidate has been widely used, but risk of abuse, dependence or psychological adverse effects make it less desirable as a long-term option.[25]

Rapid eye movement (REM) sleep behavior disorder, which can occur at any stage in the disease, is characterized by loss of atonia during REM sleep, resulting in movements ranging from twitches to punching and kicking that can potentially injure sleeping partners or the patient. Screening questionnaires are recommended and evaluation with video polysomnography of any patients suspected of having the disease. Clonazepam in low dose at bedtime is recommended first line for treatment.[3] Restless leg syndrome and periodic limb movement disorder also occur in PD at a rate that exceeds the general population. Clonazepam has also been used for the treatment of these disorders; a trial of bedtime carbidopa/levodopa can also be considered.[1]

## AUTONOMIC DYSFUNCTION SYMPTOMS
### Orthostatic Hypotension

No medications have demonstrated clear efficacy in treatment of orthostatic hypotension. Gait training, physiotherapy, and other physical interventions have also demonstrated poor long-term outcomes for this bothersome late-stage symptom.[25,30]

### Erectile Dysfunction

Small studies have suggested effective use of sildenafil for treatment of PD-related erectile dysfunction. Because of the risk of orthostatic hypotension, caution should be taken to carefully evaluate the male patient for orthostasis prior to prescribing, and there should be careful instructions for safety to prevent falls.[31]

### Constipation

Polyethylene glycol has been demonstrated to improve constipation symptoms in PD and can be used for long-term management.[25]

## Sialorrhea

Sialorrhea or drooling is a bothersome symptom that can cause significant social isolation and worsen depression and other symptoms. Glycopyrrolate was shown to be effective in short-term (1 week) use.[32] OnabotulinumtoxinA treatment demonstrated a longer-term effect, but requires training in administration and monitoring for adverse effects.[33]

## Discussion

The age of the Internet has created a unique opportunity as well as provided several challenges for providers caring for patients with PD. With access to large amounts of unfiltered data, including not only well designed studies but also sham articles published by individuals promoting particular treatments for the disease, it has become an online mine field for patients and families desperately searching for any hope. Today's clinician must develop skill in providing evidence-based answers to patients in a supportive fashion and understand that a significant number of patients will seek out complementary or alternative medicine (CAM) therapies for their PD symptoms.[34] Providers who are judgmental in their approach can cause patients to hide use of CAM and risk potential interactions with prescribed therapies. An open, supportive dialogue can encourage sharing of other more difficult symptoms, and help with developing therapeutic relationships that can help make discussions such as end-of-life care easier to facilitate with patients and families.

## REFERENCES

1. Gazewood JD, Richards DR, Clebak K. Parkinson disease: an update. Am Fam Physician 2013;87(4):267–73.
2. Fernandez H. Updates in the medical management of Parkinson disease. Cleve Clin J Med 2012;79(1):28–35.
3. Nutt JG, Wooten GF. Clinical practice. Diagnosis and initial management of Parkinson's disease. N Engl J Med 2005;353:1021–7.
4. Wright Willis A, Evanoff BA, Lian M, et al. Geographic and ethnic variation in Parkinson disease: a population-based study of US Medicare beneficiaries. Neuroepidemiology 2010;34(3):143–51.
5. Marder K, Tang MX, Mejia H, et al. Risk of Parkinson's disease among first-degree relatives: a community-based study. Neurology 1996;47(1):155–60.
6. Wider C, Ross OA, Wszolek ZK. Genetics of Parkinson disease and essential tremor. Curr Opin Neurol 2010;23(4):388–93.
7. Pezzoli G, Cereda E. Exposure to pesticides or solvents and risk of Parkinson disease. Neurology 2013;80(22):2035–41.
8. Firestone JA, Smith-Weller T, Franklin G, et al. Pesticides and risk of Parkinson disease: a population-based case-control study. Arch Neurol 2005;62(1):91.
9. Ritz B, Ascherio A, Checkoway H, et al. Pooled analysis of tobacco use and risk of Parkinson disease. Arch Neurol 2007;64(7):990–7.
10. Newman EJ, Breen K, Patterson J, et al. Accuracy of Parkinson's disease diagnosis in 610 general practice patients in the West of Scotland. Mov Disord 2009;24(16):2379–85.
11. The National Collaborating Centre for Chronic Conditions. Parkinson's disease: National clinical guideline for diagnosis and management in primary and secondary care. London: Royal College of Physicians; 2006. Available at: http://www.nice.org.uk/nicemedia/live/10984/30087/30087.pdf. Accessed March 29, 2014.

12. Bhidayasiri R, Reichmann H. Different diagnostic criteria for Parkinson disease: what are the pitfalls? J Neural Transm 2013;120(4):619–25.
13. Tolosa E, Wenning G, Poewe W. The diagnosis of Parkinson's disease. Lancet Neurol 2006;5(1):75–86.
14. Suchowersky O, Gronseth G, Perlmutter J. Practice Parameter: neuroprotective strategies and alternative therapies for Parkinson disease: an evidence-based review. Neurology 2006;66(7):976–82. Available at: https://www.aan.com/Guidelines/Home/ByTopic?topicId=17. Accessed March 29, 2014.
15. Ishihara LS, Cheesbrough A, Brayne C, et al. Estimated life expectancy of Parkinson's patients compared with the UK population. J Neurol Neurosurg Psychiatry 2007;78(12):1304–9.
16. Centers for Medicare Services EHR incentive programs meaningful use guidelines. Available at: http://www.cms.gov/Regulations-and-Guidance/Legislation/EHRIncentivePrograms/Meaningful_Use.html. Accessed March 29, 2014.
17. Miyasaki JM, Martin W, Suchowersky O, et al. Practice parameter: initiation of treatment for Parkinson's disease: an evidence-based review. Neurology 2002; 58(1):11–7.
18. Frazzitta G, Balbi P, Maestri R, et al. The beneficial role of intensive exercise on Parkinson disease progression. Am J Phys Med Rehabil 2013;92(6):523–32.
19. Grosset D, Taurah L, Burn DJ, et al. A multicentre longitudinal observational study of changes in self-reported health status in people with Parkinson's disease left untreated at diagnosis. J Neurol Neurosurg Psychiatry 2007;78(5):465–9.
20. Lees AJ, Katzenschlager R, Head J, et al. Ten-year follow-up of three different initial treatments in de-novo PD: a randomized trial. Neurology 2001;57(9): 1687–94.
21. Parkinson Study Group CALM Cohort Investigators. Long-term effect of initiating pramipexole vs levodopa in early Parkinson disease. Arch Neurol 2009;66(5): 563–70.
22. Olanow CW, Rascol O, Hauser RA, et al. A double-blind, delayed-start trial of rasagiline in Parkinson's disease. N Engl J Med 2009;361:1268–78.
23. Worth PF. How to treat Parkinson's disease in 2013. Clin Med 2013;13 (1):93–6.
24. Rodriguez-Oroz MC, Moro E, Krack P. Long-term outcomes of surgical therapies for Parkinson's disease. Mov Disord 2012;27(14):1718–28.
25. Seppi K, Weintraub D, Coelho M, et al. The movement disorder society evidence-based medicine review update: treatments for the non-motor symptoms of Parkinson's disease. Mov Disord 2011;26(Suppl 3):S42–80.
26. Emre M, Tsolaki M, Bonuccelli U, et al. Memantine for patients with Parkinson's disease dementia or dementia with Lewy bodies: a randomised, double-blind, placebo-controlled trial. Lancet Neurol 2010;9:969–77.
27. Menza M, Dobkin R, Marin H, et al. A controlled trial of antidepressants in patients with Parkinson disease and depression. Neurology 2009;72:886–92.
28. Barone P, Poewe W, Albrecht S, et al. Pramipexole for the treatment of depressive symptoms in patients with Parkinson's disease: a randomised, double-blind, placebo-controlled trial. Lancet Neurol 2010;9:573–80.
29. Lou J, Dimitrova D, Park B, et al. Using modafinil to treat fatigue in Parkinson disease: a doubleblind, placebo-controlled pilot study. Clin Neuropharmacol 2009;32:305–10.
30. Tomlinson CL, Patel S, Meek C, et al. Physiotherapy versus placebo or no intervention in Parkinson's disease. Cochrane Database Syst Rev 2012;(8):CD002817.

31. Hussain I, Brady C, Swinn M, et al. Treatment of erectile dysfunction with sildenafil citrate (Viagra) in parkinsonism due to Parkinson's disease or multiple system atrophy with observations on orthostatic hypotension. J Neurol Neurosurg Psychiatry 2001;71:371–4.
32. Arbouw M, Movig K, Koopmann M, et al. Glycopyrrolate for sialorrhea in Parkinson disease: a randomized, double-blind, crossover trial. Neurology 2010;74: 1203–7.
33. Lipp A, Trottenberg T, Schink T, et al. A randomized trial of botulinum toxin A for treatment of drooling. Neurology 2003;61:1279–81.
34. Wang Y, Xie CL, Wang WW, et al. Epidemiology of complementary and alternative medicine use in patients with Parkinson's disease. J Clin Neurosci 2013;20(8): 1062–7.

# Epilepsy
## Current Evidence-Based Paradigms for Diagnosis and Treatment

Kimberly Bates, MD

### KEYWORDS

- Epilepsy • Elderly • Traumatic brain injury • Suicide • Antiepileptic drugs

### KEY POINTS

- Epilepsy is composed of a heterogeneous group of conditions with multiple etiologies, all united by the predisposition for recurrent seizures.
- Maintain a high suspicion for epilepsy in elderly patients with neurologic complaints such as altered mental status and blackout spells, particularly those with a previous stroke.
- Young adults with epilepsy face special challenges in making the transition from pediatric to adult epilepsy care, particularly those with poorly controlled, severe epilepsy.
- Depression is one of the most frequent comorbidities seen in patients with epilepsy, and patients with depression have a higher incidence of epilepsy as compared with the general population.
- Antiepileptic medications have been associated with increased suicidal ideation and behavior; this effect was most pronounced among patients on antiepileptic drugs for the indication of epilepsy.

## NATURE OF THE PROBLEM

Epilepsy is a disease entity composed of a large number of disorders that result in recurrent seizures of varying types (**Tables 1 and 2**). Epilepsy affects about 2 million adults in the United States, or about 1% of the adult population.[1] Epilepsy can be due to a number of etiologies, including genetic predisposition, certain types of brain injury (both traumatic and anoxic), structural brain anomalies, and certain epilepsy syndromes. However, the risk for recurrent seizures is common to all patients diagnosed with epilepsy, regardless of etiology.

Department of Graduate Medical Education, 1000 Medical Center Boulevard, Lawrenceville, GA 30046, USA
*E-mail address:* kibates@gwinnettmedicalcenter.org

Prim Care Clin Office Pract 42 (2015) 217–232
http://dx.doi.org/10.1016/j.pop.2015.01.006
0095-4543/15/$ – see front matter © 2015 Elsevier Inc. All rights reserved.

**primarycare.theclinics.com**

**Table 1**
**Definition of epilepsy**

| Conceptual Definition | Operational Definition |
|---|---|
| Disease of the brain defined by: | Disease of the brain defined by: |
| Transient behaviors, signs, and/or symptoms | At least 2 unprovoked seizures >24 h apart or |
| Caused by abnormal, excessive or synchronous brain neuronal activity | 1 unprovoked seizure and a high risk of recurrence (at least 60% over the next 10 y) or |
| Due to a (presumed) underlying predisposition of the brain for such activity | Diagnosis of an epilepsy syndrome (syndrome of which epilepsy is a component) |

## CLINICAL FINDINGS
### Physical Examination

Physical examination findings depend on time of evaluation. Unless seen at the time of the seizure, examination findings are often normal. Key items of evaluation on examination include the following:

- Evidence of physical findings that may suggest a syndrome such as intellectual disability, multiple physical anomalies (such as anomalies of limb or face or asymmetry of limbs), skin findings (cutaneous neurofibromas, cafe-au-lait spots, facial angiomas, hypopigmented macules)[2]
- Evidence of neurologic insult (sensory or motor disorders, altered mental status)
- Signs of systemic illness or trauma (acute or remote)

## LABORATORY TESTING

Laboratory testing is most commonly used to rule out other conditions that can lower the seizure threshold (such as toxic ingestion, hypoglycemia, and metabolic derangements) and is most useful in the period immediately after a seizure. Serum prolactin

**Table 2**
**Common seizure types in adults**

| Types of Seizures | | Signs and Symptoms |
|---|---|---|
| Generalized | Absence | Lapse of awareness or concentration, patients do not exhibit loss of tone; no postictal confusion |
| | Myoclonic | Rapidly recurrent, bilateral shocklike jerks to the face, trunk, and extremities, with or without loss of consciousness |
| | Tonic-clonic | Associated with loss of consciousness; may initially present with premonitory symptoms, such as irritability or feeling of fear; followed by postictal period characterized by altered mental status (confusion, drowsiness, irritability), headache, and generalized myalgias |
| Partial | Simple | Focal rhythmic contractions that may result in limb jerking, head turning, and so forth without loss of consciousness or awareness |
| | Complex | Often accompanied by automatisms (lip smacking, chewing); loss of consciousness preceded by aura, such as altered emotion, sensation, or movement; as with simple partial seizures, are focal in nature and presenting symptom depends on location |

can be elevated immediately after a seizure, but must be compared with a baseline serum level to be diagnostically useful.

## SPECIAL CONSIDERATIONS
### Elderly

Among adults, elderly patients (age>65) have the highest incidence of new-onset epilepsy.[3] However, the diagnosis of epilepsy in elderly individuals can be difficult for several reasons. Complex partial seizures are the most common form of epilepsy in elderly patients, yet patients are unlikely to describe or exhibit aura or automatisms, which are typical signs of complex partial seizures in younger patients.[3] Elderly patients may also present with atypical manifestations of epilepsy, including longer postictal confusion.[3] On average, there is a delay of 1.7 years from the time of symptom onset to the diagnosis of epilepsy in elderly patients, in part due to the complexity of diagnosis in the elderly.[3] A high index of suspicion for epilepsy is warranted in elderly patients with presenting symptoms of altered mental status, confusion, or blackout spells, particularly in those with risk factors for epilepsy (**Table 3**).

### Transition of Youth with Epilepsy to Adult Care

Youth with epilepsy, particularly poorly controlled epilepsy, require transition to adult neurology care as they age. Many youth with epilepsy have multiple comorbidities associated with their epilepsy, such as congenital disease; mental health issues, such as depression, anxiety and attention-deficit/hyperactivity disorder; and intellectual disabilities such as autism. Baca, et al. have shown that youth with active seizures suffer worse quality of life in terms of physical and psychosocial function in comparison to youth with epilepsy in remission.[4] In addition, young adults with childhood epilepsy may be at further risk of comorbidities due to duration of AED usage. Providers who will assume epilepsy management for young adults must remain as diligent in screening for co-morbidities and treating epilepsy related complications in these patients as they would for much older patients. In addition, these patients may require greater usage of medical services than their age alone would suggest, given the issues mentioned above. Adult providers will need to become comfortable with congenital medical conditions associated with epilepsy, as well as treatment of patients with intellectual disabilities in order to properly serve this demographic.

### Traumatic Brain Injury

Patients with traumatic brain injury are at significant risk of epilepsy. In addition, the severity of traumatic brain injury (TBI) is positively associated with risk of posttraumatic epilepsy.[5] Posttraumatic epilepsy tends to refer to late-onset seizures (those occurring more than 1 week after TBI). Studies of both military and civilian patients report higher incidence of posttraumatic epilepsy in patients with early posttraumatic seizures, multiple comorbidities (including depression), and severe TBI.[6] Studies also

| Table 3 | |
|---|---|
| **Risk factors for new-onset epilepsy in elderly individuals** | |
| Cerebrovascular Disease (Stroke)[a] | Dementia |
| Head trauma | Brain tumor |
| Inflammatory disorders | Alzheimer disease |

[a] Most common cause of new-onset epilepsy in elderly persons.

have noted the risk of epilepsy diagnosis is higher in the immediate post-TBI period but never declines to zero.[7] A longitudinal study of Danish children and young adults who sustained a TBI noted an increased risk of epilepsy in those who sustained a TBI at any time during childhood, with the highest risk for those who sustained a severe brain injury before age 5 or after age 15.[7] The risk of development of epilepsy persisted through 10 years post-TBI in this study. Thus, the index of suspicion for the development of epilepsy in patients with severe TBI should remain high, even as far as 10 years after injury.

### Women of Childbearing Age

Women with epilepsy face several challenges, particularly as it relates to seizure control and treatment. Menstruating women may have increased seizure activity around menstrual cycles (catamenial seizures), causing increased difficulty with seizure control. In addition, many antiepileptic drugs (AEDs) have significant teratogenic effects, particularly valproic acid and phenytoin. Newer AEDs have fewer data on use in pregnancy. For some women, this becomes a choice between risking worsening seizure control and risking teratogenicity during pregnancy. For women who do not wish to have children, contraceptive options had been limited previously. AEDs decrease the activity of oral contraceptives, making unintended pregnancy more likely. There is also evidence of decreased efficacy of certain AEDs (those with P450 metabolism) when used with oral contraceptives, which may lead to breakthrough seizures. In the era of long-acting reversible contraceptives (LARCs), such as intrauterine devices and implantable progestin-delivering devices, there are now more acceptable options for contraception in women with epilepsy. However, more study is needed to ensure efficacy with LARCs and AEDs in these women.

### Comorbidities

Patients with epilepsy have a high incidence of comorbidities. According to the National Health Interview Survey, more than 70% of adults with a diagnosis of epilepsy have 3 or more nonpsychiatric comorbidities, compared with fewer than 50% of adults with no history of epilepsy.[8] Adults with epilepsy also report higher rates of smoking and physical inactivity and have a higher rate of obesity than the general population.[9] All of these factors increase the complexity of caring for adults with epilepsy. The EPIC Survey (Epilepsy Comorbidities and Health) found neuropsychiatric conditions (such as depression, anxiety, and sleep disorders) and pain disorders (such as migraine and chronic pain) to be the most prevalent comorbidities among adults with self-reported epilepsy.[10] Significant association exists between type of seizure disorder and neuropsychiatric comorbidity. Depression is the most commonly reported psychiatric disorder in both youth and adults with epilepsy, and is most strongly associated with partial epilepsy.[10–12] Depressive symptoms have been well described in adults, and seem to be independent of seizure frequency or other factors that may be associated with chronic illness.[10] A recent meta-analysis on depression and epilepsy reported on the suggestion of a bidirectional influence of depression on the development of epilepsy and its treatment.[13]

Quality of life in youth and adults with epilepsy is also affected. In children with epilepsy, quality of life measured by the Child Health Questionnaire 9 years after diagnosis was significantly lower in children with recurrent seizures (defined as seizures within the past 12 months), particularly in the domains of physical function, social limitations due to physical issues, behavior, and family activities.[4] Adults with epilepsy have similar declines of quality of life related to seizure frequency. In a meta-analysis of studies on health care quality of life in adults with epilepsy, Taylor et al.

found that health care quality of life was negatively associated with seizure frequency and severity, presence of comorbidities, and history of depression and anxiety.[14] Given the prevalence of depression and other comorbidities in adults with epilepsy, this review suggests that assessing quality of life in all patients with epilepsy should be part of whole-person–oriented epilepsy management.

## TREATMENT

Table 4 lists the AEDs that are approved by the Food and Drug Administration (FDA) in the United States for treatment of epilepsy by class and indication. Many of these agents are newer (FDA approved in the past 5 years), and are approved only as an adjunct for patients who do not achieve seizure control on standard therapies, such as valproic acid, phenytoin, levetiracetam, or lamotrigine.

## SUICIDE RISK WITH ANTIEPILEPTIC DRUGS

In 2009, the FDA issued a warning about suicidal ideation and behavior in patients on AEDs (both as monotherapy and adjunctive therapy). This resulted in the issuance of a black box warning for AEDs on suicidality risk. The warning stemmed from the FDA Statistical Review and Evaluation of Antiepileptic Drugs and Suicidality, May 23, 2008,[15] which was a primary analysis of 199 pooled placebo-controlled AED medication trials, consisting of more than 27,000 patients with AED exposure. The analysis showed an odds ratio of 2.92 for suicidal behavior (characterized by completed suicide, suicide attempt, or preparatory acts toward imminent suicidal behavior) compared with placebo. Overall, this appeared to be a class effect, and persisted despite controlling for mechanism of action, age, race, or gender. Although studies in this analysis included patients who were on AEDs for reasons other than epilepsy, patients treated for epilepsy had the highest odds ratio at 3.53 for suicidal ideation and behavior compared with placebo. This amounted to 2.4 additional patients per 1000 treated patients with a suicidal event related to AED drug exposure.

## NONADHERENCE TO ANTIEPILEPTIC DRUG THERAPY

One of the greatest challenges to seizure control in patients with epilepsy is the problem of nonadherence to therapy. In a survey of patients and physicians, Hovinga and colleagues[16] found a nonadherence rate approximating 30%. Perhaps not surprisingly, patients with self-reported nonadherence had worsening seizure control, decreased quality-of-life scores and decreased productivity compared with patients with better reported adherence. Those with lower self-reported adherence also had greater utilization of resources (more emergency department [ED] visits, more physician office visits).[16] Given that patients with an epilepsy diagnosis have been shown to exert greater economic burden to the health care system,[17] one could assume nonadherence to therapy may represent a significant component of that burden. Notably, the authors of the RANSOM study, which looked at adherence and health care utilization among a large cohort of more than 30,000 patients with epilepsy, saw an increase in health care utilization and health costs among patients who were nonadherent compared with those who were adherent.[18] When providers are confronted with worsening seizure control or with patients with frequent ED usage or hospitalizations related to epilepsy, nonadherence to therapy should be at the top of the differential during assessment of efficacy of current antiepileptic regimen.

**Table 4**
**Antiepileptic medications approved by the Food and Drug Administration for use in the United States**

| | Generic Name | Mechanism of Action | How Supplied | Dosing | Adjustments in Renal/Hepatic Impairment | Side Effects, Contraindications, Monitoring |
|---|---|---|---|---|---|---|
| **Class: Hydantoins** | | | | | | |
| Generalized tonic-clonic or complex partial seizure (CPS) | Ethotoin Brand name: Peganone | Stabilizes the seizure threshold and prevents spread of seizure activity (hydantoin) | Oral 250-mg tablet | Initial: <1000 mg daily Maintenance: 2000–3000 mg daily | None/ contraindicated in patients with hepatic abnormalities | Blood dyscrasias, systemic lupus erythematosus-like syndrome, Stevens-Johnson syndrome |
| Status epilepticus | Fosphenytoin Brand name: Cerebyx | Stabilizing neuronal membranes and increasing efflux or decreasing influx of sodium ions across cell membranes in the motor cortex during generation of nerve impulses | IM or IV | Loading (status): 15–20 phenytoin sodium equivalents (PE)/kg at 100–150 mg PE/min Loading (nonemergent): 10–20 PE/kg over 30 min Maintenance: 4–6 PE/kg/d in divided doses | No/No | Blood dyscrasias, hypotension, cardiac arrhythmias, severe dermatologic reactions (toxic epidermal necrolysis, Stevens-Johnson syndrome, DRESS-Drug Reaction with Eosinophilia and Systemic Symptoms), purple glove syndrome (discoloration with edema and pain of distal limb) Therapeutic range: 10–20 μg/mL Toxic: >30 μg/mL Lethal: >100 μg/mL |

**Class: Miscellaneous**

| | | | | | | |
|---|---|---|---|---|---|---|
| Partial seizures, adjunct | Ezogabine Brand name: Potiga | Binds to voltage-gated potassium channels, stabilizing the channels in the open formation to regulate neuronal excitability and suppress epileptiform activity | Oral 50, 200, 300, 400 mg tablets | Initial: 100 mg 3 times daily Maintenance: 750 mg daily in divided doses | Yes/Yes | Skin discoloration (blue, gray-blue, or brown), neuropsychiatric disorders, such as psychotic symptoms and hallucinations, retinal abnormalities that may progress to vision loss (recommend screening eye examination every 6 mo), urinary retention |
| Partial seizures with complex symptom-ology (such as temporal lobe epilepsy), generalized tonic-clonic seizure, mixed seizure patterns | Carbamazepine Brand name: Tegretol | Limiting influx of sodium ions across cell membranes by decreasing temporal stimulation | Oral 100, 200 and 300 mg tablets, 12 h extended-release tablets | Initial: 400 mg/d in 2 divided doses Maintenance: usual 800–1200 mg daily, maximum 1600 mg/d | Yes/use with caution in hepatic impairment | Blood dyscrasias, toxic epidermal necrolysis, and Stevens-Johnson syndrome (increased in patients with HLA-B*1502, almost exclusively seen in patients of Asian ancestry), hyponatremia, DRESS, psychosis |

(continued on next page)

**Table 4**
**(continued)**

| | Generic Name | Mechanism of Action | How Supplied | Dosing | Adjustments in Renal/Hepatic Impairment | Side Effects, Contraindications, Monitoring |
|---|---|---|---|---|---|---|
| Partial seizure, adjunct | Eslicarbazepine Brand name: Aptiom | Thought to involve inhibition of voltage-gated sodium channels | Oral 200, 400 and 600 mg tablets | Initial: 400 mg once daily × 1 wk Maintenance: 800–1200 mg once daily | Yes/No (not recommended in severe hepatic impairment, however) | SJS, cognitive symptoms (memory impairment, amnesia, slowness of thought, aphasia), coordination abnormalities (ataxia, vertigo, balance disorder), visual changes, mild to moderate elevations in transaminases (>3× ULN), hyponatremia and hypochloremia, DRESS |
| Partial seizures, monotherapy or adjunctive; adjunctive treatment for seizures secondary to Lennox-Gaustaut syndrome | Felbamate Brand name: Felbato | Weak inhibitory effects on GABA-receptor binding | Oral 400 and 600 mg tablets, 600 mg/5 mL suspension | Initial: 1200 mg/d in divided doses 3 to 4 times daily Maintenance: up 3600 mg/d in divided doses 3 to 4 times daily | Yes/contraindicated | Aplastic anemia, hepatic failure |

| Partial seizures | Gabapentin Brand name: Gralise, Neurontin | GABA analog that appears to bind to voltage-gated calcium channels and modulate release of excitatory neurotransmitters that participate in epileptogenesis | Oral 100, 300, 400, 600 and 800 mg tablets, 250 mg/mL oral solution | Initial: 300 mg 3 times daily Maintenance: 900–1800 mg daily in divided doses 3 times daily | Yes/No | DRESS, neuropsychiatric effects, such as emotional lability, aggressive behaviors, concentration problems, and hyperkinesia |
|---|---|---|---|---|---|---|
| Partial seizures, monotherapy and adjunct | Lacosamide Brand name: Vimpat | Stabilizes hyperexcitable neuronal membranes and inhibits repetitive neuronal firing by enhancing slow inactivation of sodium channels | Oral, IV 50,100, 150 and 200 mg tablet 10 mg/mL oral solution 200 mg/20 mL IV solution | Monotherapy Initial: 100 mg twice daily Maintenance: 150–200 mg twice daily Adjunctive Therapy Initial: 50 mg twice daily Maintenance: 100–200 mg twice daily | Yes/Yes | QT interval prolongation, heart block, ataxia, DRESS, vision disturbances |
| Partial seizures, generalized tonic-clonic, Lennox-Gastaut (all adjunctive) | Lamotrigine Brand name: Lamictal | Inhibits release of glutamate and inhibits voltage-sensitive sodium channels, stabilizing neuronal membranes | Oral IR: 2, 5, 25, 50, 100, 150, 200 mg tablets ER: 25, 50, 100, 200, 250 and 300 mg tablets | Initial: titrate up slowly from 25 mg every other day to every day. Add 25–50 mg every 1–2 wk Maintenance: 100–500 mg daily (based on primary anticonvulsant in regimen) | No/Yes | Aseptic meningitis, blood dyscrasias, DRESS, SJS, TEN, angioedema |

(continued on next page)

**Table 4**
*(continued)*

| Generic Name | Mechanism of Action | How Supplied | Dosing | Adjustments in Renal/Hepatic Impairment | Side Effects, Contraindications, Monitoring |
|---|---|---|---|---|---|
| Myoclonic seizures, partial seizures, tonic-clonic seizures | | | | | |
| Levetiracetam Brand name: Keppra | Unknown but possible mechanisms include inhibition of voltage-dependent calcium channels, facilitation of GABA-ergic inhibitory transmission | Oral/IV IR: 250, 500, 750 and 1000 mg ER:500 and 750 mg IV: 500 mg/5 mL, 500 mg/100 mL, 1000 mg/100 mL, 1500 mg/100 mL | Initial: 500 mg twice daily Maintenance: 1500–3000 mg twice daily Status epilepticus: 1000–3000 mg IV over 15 min | Yes/No (unless severe hepatic impairment and renal impairment) | Impaired coordination, weakness, somnolence, TEN, SJS, anemia, eosinophilia, lymphocytosis, psychiatric symptoms, including psychosis, paranoia, hallucinations, emotional lability |
| Partial seizures, monotherapy or adjunct | | | | | |
| Oxcarbazepine Brand name: Trileptal, Oxtellar XR | Blocks voltage-gated sodium channels, stabilizing hyperexcited neuronal membranes | Oral IR: 150, 300 and 600 mg ER: 150, 300 and 600 mg 300 mg/5 mL oral solution | Initial: 600 mg/d (in 2 divided doses for IR) Maintenance: 1200 mg/d adjunctive therapy, 2400 mg/d monotherapy | Yes/No | Blood dyscrasias, osteopenia, osteoporosis, cognitive symptoms, including difficulty with concentration, speech or language problems, somnolence and coordination difficulties, DRESS, hyponatremia, hypothyroidism, hepatic dysfunction |

| Indication | Drug | Mechanism | Route/Form | Dosing | | Side Effects |
|---|---|---|---|---|---|---|
| Partial seizures, adjunct | Perampanel Brand name: Fycompa | Noncompetitive antagonist of the glutamate receptor on postsynaptic neurons | Oral 2, 4, 6, 8, 10 and 12 mg tablets | Initial: 2-4 mg once daily at bedtime Maintenance: 8-12 mg once daily at bedtime | No/Yes | Dizziness, fatigue, neuropsychiatric effects, such as aggression, irritability, homicidal thoughts |
| Partial seizure, adjunct | Pregabalin Brand name: Lyrica | Inhibits neurotransmitter release by binding to voltage-gated calcium channels | Oral 25, 50, 75, 100, 150, 200, 225, and 300 mg capsules 20 mg/mL liquid | Initial: 150 mg daily in divided doses Maintenance: up to 600 mg daily in divided doses | Yes/No | Angioedema, dizziness and somnolence, hypersensitivity, peripheral edema, thrombocytopenia, rhabdomyolysis, visual disturbances, weight gain |
| Generalized tonic-clonic, partial, monotherapy and adjunct | Primidone Brand Name: Mysoline | Decreases neuron excitability, active metabolite is phenobarbital | Oral 50 and 250 mg tablets | Initial: 100–125 mg daily, titrating up every 3 d to 3 times daily Maintenance: 750–1000 mg/d in 3 divided doses | No/No | CNS depression |
| Partial seizure, adjunct | Tiagabine Brand name: Gabitril | Enhances GABA activity | Oral 2, 4, 12, and 16 mg tablets | Initial: 4 mg once daily Maintenance: 32–56 mg/d in 2–4 divided doses | No/No | CNS depression, TEN, SJS |

(continued on next page)

**Table 4**
*(continued)*

| | Generic Name | Mechanism of Action | How Supplied | Dosing | Adjustments in Renal/Hepatic Impairment | Side Effects, Contraindications, Monitoring |
|---|---|---|---|---|---|---|
| Partial seizure, generalized tonic-clonic seizure, monotherapy and adjunct, Lennox-Gastaut, adjunct only | Topiramate Brand name: Topamax, Topiragen, Trokendi XR, Qudexy XR | Blocks voltage-dependent sodium channels in neurons, enhances GABA activity | Oral IR: 25, 50, 100, and 200 mg tablets; 15 and 25 mg capsule sprinkle ER: 25, 50, 100, 150, 200 mg capsule and capsule sprinkles | Initial: 25 mg 1–2 times daily, titrating up weekly Maintenance: 400 mg/d, in 2 divided doses for IR | Yes/No | Cognitive dysfunction, hyperammonemia/encephalopathy, metabolic acidosis due to inhibition of carbonic anhydrase, oligohydrosis and hyperthermia, angle-closure glaucoma, kidney stone |
| Absence seizure, CPS, combination types that include absence seizures monotherapy and adjunctive therapy | Valproic acid derivatives Brand name: Depacon, Depakene, Depakote, Stavzor | Increases neuronal availability of GAVA | Oral IR: 250 mg DR: 125, 250, 500 mg ER: 250, 500 mg Sprinkle capsule: 125 mg Liquid: 250 mg/5 mL | Initial: 10–15 mg/kg/d in 1–3 divided doses Maintenance: up to 60 mg/kg/d in divided doses | Yes/Not recommended for use in hepatic disease | Brain atrophy, CNS depression, hepatic failure, hyperammonemia/encephalopathy, hypothermia, DRESS, pancreatitis, thrombocytopenia Serum monitoring Therapeutic Range: 20–100 µg/mL Toxic: >100–200 µg/mL |
| Refractory CPS, adjunct | Vigabatrin Brand name: Sabril | Irreversibly inhibits GABA transaminase, increasing GABA in the brain | Oral 500 mg tablet or packet | Initial: 500 mg twice daily Maintenance: up to 1500 mg twice daily | Yes/No | Permanent vision loss, anemia, somnolence, peripheral neuropathy, edema, weight gain |

| Indication | Drug / Brand name | Mechanism of action | Formulation | Dosage | Not recommended/ | Adverse effects |
|---|---|---|---|---|---|---|
| Partial seizure, adjunct | Zonisamide Brand name: Zonegran | Unknown but thought to stabilize neuronal membranes through action at sodium and calcium channels | Oral 25, 50, and 100 mg capsules | Initial: 100 mg/d Maintenance: up to 400 mg/d | No | Psychiatric symptoms, fatigue, sedation, metabolic acidosis, kidney stones, sulfonamide reactions |
| **Class: Succinimides** | | | | | | |
| Absence seizures, monotherapy | Ethosuximide Brand name: Zarontin | Depresses nerve transmission in motor cortex, increases seizure threshold through unknown mechanism | Oral 250 mg capsule 250 mg/5 mL oral solution | Initial: 500 mg/d Maintenance: up to 1500 mg/d in divided doses | No/No | Blood dyscrasias, CNS depression, SJS, lupus (SLE) |
| Refractory absence seizures | Methsuximide Brand name: Celontin | Depresses nerve transmission in motor cortex, increases seizure threshold through unknown mechanism | Oral 300 mg capsule | Initial: 300 mg/d Maintenance: up to 1200 mg/d in 2–4 divided doses | No/No | Blood dyscrasias, CNS depression, SLE |
| Lennox-Gastaut syndrome, adjunct | Rufinamide Brand name: Banzel | Prolongs inactive state of sodium channels, limiting repetitive firing of sodium-dependent action potentials | Oral 200 and 400 mg tablets 40 mg/mL suspension | Initial: 400–800 mg/d in 2 divided doses Maintenance: up to 3200 mg/d in 2 divided doses | No/Use with caution | Shortening of QT interval (contraindicated in patients with familial short QT syndrome), cognitive symptoms, and coordination abnormalities, DRESS, SJS |

(continued on next page)

**Table 4**
**(continued)**

| Generic Name | Mechanism of Action | How Supplied | Dosing | Adjustments in Renal/Hepatic Impairment | Side Effects, Contraindications, Monitoring |
|---|---|---|---|---|---|
| **Class: Barbiturates** | | | | | |
| Generalized tonic-clonic seizures, partial seizures, status epilepticus | Phenobarbital | Decreases neuron excitability, depresses sensory cortex | Oral 15, 16.2, 30, 32.4, 60, 64.8, 97.2, and 100 mg tablets 20 mg/5 mL elixir IV: 65 mg/mL solution | Maintenance: 50–100 mg 2 or 3 times daily Status epilepticus: 20 mg/kg, may repeat with additional 5–10 mg/kg | Yes/No: use with caution | CNS depression, hypotension (IV), respiratory depression, paradoxic stimulatory response |
| Refractory status epilepticus | Pentobarbital Brand name: Nembutal | Reduces brain metabolism and cerebral blood flow, decreases neuron excitability | IV 50 mg/mL | Initial: 10–15 mg/kg loading dose Maintenance infusion: 0.5–1 mg/kg/h, adjusted to maintain burst suppression pattern on EEG | No/No | Requires endotracheal intubation for airway protection |

*Abbreviations:* CNS, central nervous system; CPS, complex partial seizures; DR, delayed release; DRESS, drug rash with eosinophilia and systemic symptoms; EEG, electroencephalogram; ER, extended release; IM, intramuscular; IR, immediate release; IV, intravenous; SJS, Stevens Johnson Syndrome; SLE, systemic lupus erythematosus; TEN, toxic epidermal necrolysis; ULN, upper limit of normal.
Mechanism of action, dosing information, side effects, contraindications and monitoring information. *Adapted from LexiComp drug reference 1978–2014.* Available at: http://online.lexi.com/.

## SUMMARY

Epilepsy is a heterogeneous and complication condition, with significant morbidity and impacts on quality of life. Several special populations, including the elderly, women of child-bearing age, those with posttraumatic brain injury, and young adults with active childhood epilepsy require special consideration. Challenges that physicians face in diagnosing and treating patients with epilepsy include maintaining strong diagnostic suspicion, managing co-morbidities, and identifying adverse effects of AEDs, including potential suicidality. Although treatment of epilepsy with newer AEDs has expanded the therapeutic options for patients with epilepsy, nonadherence to AED therapy continues to be one of the greatest challenges in caring for those with epilepsy. Because of the myriad of complications and considerations required to manage these patients, primary care providers should partner with epileptologists to manage patients with epilepsy long-term. However, the primary care provider has a unique opportunity to surveil for comorbidities, such as mental health disorders (particularly suicidal ideation) and pain disorders (including migraine), and to assess for impact of disease on overall quality of life.

## REFERENCES

1. Centers for Disease Control and Prevention (CDC). Epiepsy in Adults and Access to Care - United States, 2010. MMWR Mab Mortal Wkly Rep 2012;61(45): 909–13.
2. Alexopoulos A, Wijdicks E, Sisson S. Epilepsy in adults. First Consult. Elsevier; 2011.
3. Pugh M, Knoefel J, Mortensen E, et al. New-onset epilepsy risk factors in older veterans. J Am Geriatr Soc 2009;57(2):237–42.
4. Baca C, Vickrey B, Vassar S, et al. Seizure recency and quality of life in adolescents with childhood-onset epilepsy. Epilepsy Behav 2012;23:47–51.
5. Ferguson P, Smith G, Wannamakr B, et al. A population based study of risk of epilepsy after hospitalization for traumatic brain injury. Epilepsia 2010;51(5): 891–8.
6. Lowenstein D. Epilepsy after head injury: an overview. Epilepsia 2009;50(Suppl. 2): 4–9.
7. Christensen J, Pedersen M, Pedersen C, et al. Long-term risk of epilepsy after traumatic brain injury in children and young adults: a population-based cohort study. Lancet 2009;373:1105–10.
8. Centers for Disease Control and Prevention (CDC). Comorbidity in adults with epilepsy—United States, 2010. MMWR Morb Mortal Wkly Rep 2013;62(43):849–53.
9. Centers for Disease Control and Prevention (CDC). Epilepsy surveillance among adults—19 states, Behavioral Risk Factor Surveillance System, 2005. MMWR Surveill Summ 2008;57(6):1–20.
10. Ottman R, Lipton R, Ettinger AB, et al. Comorbidities of epilepsy: results from the Epilepsy Comorbidities and Health (EPIC) survey. Epilepsia 2011;52(2):308–15.
11. Stevanovic D, Jancic J, Lakic A. The impact of depression and anxiety disorder symptoms on the health-related quality of life of children and adolescents with epilepsy. Epilepsia 2011;52(8):e75–8.
12. Ekinci O, Titus J, Rodopman A, et al. Depression and anxiety in children and adolescents with epilepsy: prevalence, risk factors, and treatment. Epilepsy Behav 2009;14:8–18.
13. Fiest K, Dykeman J, Patten SB, et al. Depression in epilepsy: a meta-analysis and systematic review. Neurology 2013;80(6):590–9.

14. Taylor RS, Sander J, Taylor RJ, et al. Predictors of health-related quality of life and costs in adults with epilepsy: a systematic review. Epilepsia 2011;52(12): 2168–80.
15. Levenson M, Rochester C, Mentari E, et al. Statistical review and evaluation: anti-epileptic drugs and suicidality. US Food and Drug Administration. Center for Drug Evaluation and Research. Office of Translational Sciences, Office of Biostatistics. May 23, 2008.
16. Hovinga C, Asato M, Manjunath R, et al. Association of non-adherence to antiepileptic drugs and seizures, quality of life, and productivity: survey of patients with epilepsy and physicians. Epilepsy Behav 2008;13:316–22.
17. Ivanova J, Birnbaum H, Kidolezi Y, et al. Economic burden of epilepsy among the privately insured in the US. Pharmacoeconomics 2010;28(8):675–85.
18. Faught R, Weiner J, Guerin A, et al. Impact of nonadherence to antiepileptic drugs on health care utilization and costs: findings from the RANSOM study. Epilepsia 2009;50(3):501–9.

# Diagnosis and Management of Migraines and Migraine Variants

Tomia Palmer Harmon, MD

## KEYWORDS

- Migraine • Treatment • Medications • NSAIDs • Triptans • Antiemetics

## KEY POINTS

- Migraine headache is a neurologic disorder that has been widely studied.
- There are several treatment options available for mild to severe migraine headache.
- Adults with mild to moderate migraine headache and vomiting should add an antiemetic to their regimen; children and adults with moderate to severe migraine should try parenteral therapies like sumatriptan nasal spray.
- Relaxation training and cognitive–behavioral therapy have a role in nonpharmacologic treatment options; surgical removal of trigger points has been found to be effective.

## INTRODUCTION

A migraine headache is a complex brain event that takes place over hours to days.[1] Migraine headache takes on many different forms and levels of severity. Additionally, migraine affects adults as well as children. Patients who may require preventive therapy include patients with more than 4 migraine headaches per month, patients with migraine headaches that last for more than 12 hours, and those who feel that migraine accounts for a significant amount of their total disability.[2] Other patients who might require preventive therapy are those who have a resultant neurologic deficit secondary to migraine or those for whom the cost of acute therapy is prohibitive. The same symptomatology that leads to preventive therapy in adults applies to children. However, some patients are well-controlled with acute therapies. This article highlights treatment options for acute migraine in children and adults.

## PATIENT EVALUATION OVERVIEW

The diagnosis of migraine headache is made based on patient history of headaches that fit a set of diagnostic criteria (**Box 1**). Criteria set forth by

Department of Clinical Education, Georgia Campus, Philadelphia College of Osteopathic Medicine, 625 Old Peachtree Road, Northwest, Suwanee, GA 30024, USA
*E-mail address:* tomiaha@pcom.edu

Prim Care Clin Office Pract 42 (2015) 233–241
http://dx.doi.org/10.1016/j.pop.2015.01.003
0095-4543/15/$ – see front matter © 2015 Elsevier Inc. All rights reserved.

**Box 1**
**Diagnostic criteria for migraine**

*Migraine without aura*

A. At least 5 attacks fulfilling criteria B–D

B. Headache attacks lasting 4–72 hours (untreated or unsuccessfully treated)

C. Headache has ≥2 of the following characteristics:

Unilateral location

Pulsating quality

Moderate or severe pain intensity

Aggravation by or causing avoidance of routine physical activity (eg, walking or climbing stairs)

D. During headache ≥1 of the following:

Nausea, vomiting, or both

Photophobia and phonophobia

E. Not better accounted for by another ICHD-3 diagnosis

*Migraine with aura*

A. At least 2 attacks fulfilling criterion B and C

B. One or more of the following fully reversible aura symptoms:

Visual

Sensory

Speech and/or language

Motor

Brainstem

Retinal

C. At least 2 of the following 4 characteristics:

At least 1 aura symptom spreads gradually over ≥5 minutes, and/or ≥2 symptoms occur in succession

Each individual aura symptom lasts 5–60 minutes

At least 1 aura symptom is unilateral

The aura is accompanied, or followed within 60 minutes, by headache

D. Not better accounted for by another ICHD-3 diagnosis, and transient ischemic attack has been excluded

*Migraine with typical aura*

A. At least 2 attacks fulfilling criteria B–D

B. Aura consisting of visual, sensory, and/or speech/language symptoms, each fully reversible, but no motor, brainstem, or retinal symptoms

C. At least 2 of the following 4 characteristics:

At least 1 aura symptom spreads gradually over ≥5 minutes, and/or ≥2 symptoms occur in succession

Each individual aura symptom lasts 5–60 minutes

At least 1 aura symptom is unilateral

The aura is accompanied, or followed within 60 minutes, by headache

D. Not better accounted for by another ICHD-3 diagnosis, and transient ischemic attack has been excluded

*Features of migraine in children*

Attacks may last 2–72 hours

Headache is more often bilateral than in adults; an adult pattern of unilateral pain usually emerges in late adolescence or early adulthood

Occipital headache is rare and raises diagnostic caution for structural lesions

Photophobia and phonophobia may be inferred by behavior in young children

*Abbreviation:* ICHD-3, International Classification of Headache Disorders, 3rd edition.
   *Adapted from* Headache Classification Committee of the International Headache Society (HIS). The international classification of headache disorders, 3rd edition (beta version). Cephalalgia 2013;33:629.

the International Headache Society for acute migraine without aura are as follows[3]:

1. More than 5 attacks of the same type headache, lasting 4 to 72 hours
2. Headache (2 criteria must apply):
   a. Unilateral
   b. Throbbing or pulsating
   c. Aggravated by activity
   d. Moderate to severe intensity
3. Associated symptoms ($\geq$1):
   a. Nausea or vomiting
   b. Phonophobia or photophobia

Patients might also have other symptoms that are listed in the diagnostic criteria for migraine with aura, migraine with typical aura, and migraine in children. Those criteria are listed in **Box 1**.

The International Headache Society also defines migraine as either episodic or chronic. Episodic migraine occurs on fewer than 15 days of the month for fewer than 3 months. Chronic migraine occurs on more than 15 days of the month for more than 3 months.

Children with migraine headaches may not be able to express adequately their symptomatology. Neurologists suggest that children use headache drawings to try to illustrate their pain. Illustrations showing features like pounding pain, nausea/vomiting, and photophobia have been found to be 92.1% sensitive and 82.7% specific, with a positive predictive value of 87.1% for migraine.[4]

Studies have shown that the diagnostic criteria may have decreased sensitivity when children are seen in the emergency department. Therefore, a set of criteria have been proposed for the diagnosis of children in the emergency department.[5] Four of the 6 criteria listed below should be met:

- Moderate to severe episode of impaired daily activities
- Focal localization of headache
- Pulsatile description
- Nausea or vomiting or abdominal pain
- Photophobia or phonophobia or avoidance of light and noise
- Symptoms increasing with activity or resolving by rest.

Treatment of migraine is just as complex as diagnosis. There are pharmacologic and nonpharmacologic treatment options, as well as combination therapies and surgical treatment options.

## PHARMACOLOGIC TREATMENT OPTIONS

Treatment of migraine headache should mirror the severity of migraine and symptoms. A randomized, controlled, parallel-group clinical trial conducted by the Disability in Strategies Study Group in 13 countries has shown that early treatment of migraine with a large dose of medication deemed better clinical results compared with a stepwise approach.[6,7] The study found that headache response at 2 hours across 6 attacks was 52.7% in the stratified care treatment group versus 40.6% in the step care across attacks group.

Intensity of medication care should be linked to severity of symptoms.[2] A patient who has mild to moderate migraines without nausea and vomiting should be given prescriptions for nonsteroidal anti-inflammatory drugs (NSAIDs), acetaminophen, or combination analgesics. An antiemetic should be added to the NSAIDs, acetaminophen, or combination analgesic in the patient with mild to moderate migraines with nausea and vomiting. Patients with moderate to severe migraines without nausea and vomiting should be started on triptans or a combination of sumatriptan-naproxen (Treximet); those patients with nausea and vomiting in the setting of a moderate to severe migraine can try medications like nasal sumatriptan (Imitrex), parenteral dihydroergotamine (Migranal, D.H.E. 45), and antiemetics that can be given by a nonoral route (**Table 1**).[2]

For treatment of mild to moderate migraine, a review of UpToDate shows that the following NSAIDs have been found to be effective in the treatment of migraine headache in randomized, placebo-controlled trials[8]:

- Aspirin (Ecotrin), 650 to 1000 mg
- Ibuprofen (Motrin), 400 to 1200 mg
- Naproxen (Aleve; Naprosyn), 750 to 1250 mg
- Diclofenac (Voltaren, Cataflam), 50 to 100 mg
- Diclofenac epolamine (Flector Patch), 65 mg
- Acetaminophen (Tylenol), 1000 mg
- Acetaminophen–aspirin–caffeine (Excedrin), 2 extra-strength tablets

Treximet (a proprietary formulation of sumatriptan 85 mg and naproxen 500 mg) has been recommended for patients who do not respond well to monotherapy. A randomized, placebo-controlled trial found that sumatriptan–naproxen was effective at reducing headache pain, photophobia, and phonophobia. A dose of naproxen 550 mg (over-the-counter formulation) and a single oral sumatriptan can be given to patients if cost is prohibitive.[9]

Metoclopramide (Reglan) at a dose of 10 mg antiemetic is used as an adjunctive therapy for mild to moderate migraine and has been found to decrease nausea and vomiting.[10] Metoclopramide is used normally only in children in the emergency setting or when the child has extended migraine.

Triptans have been found to be effective in the treatment of moderate to severe migraine headache.[2] The oral triptans available to treatment of migraine headache without nausea and vomiting are as follows:

- Eletriptan (Relpax), 40 mg
- Naratriptan (Amerge), 2.5 mg
- Rizatriptan (Maxalt), 5 or 10 mg
- Sumatriptan (Imitrex), 100 mg
- Zolmitriptan (Zomig), 2.5, 5, or 10 mg

But what happens if your patient has moderate to severe migraines and has concurrent nausea and vomiting? There are parenteral medications that can be used for treatment. Parenteral sumatriptan (Imitrex Injection, Imitrex Nasal Spray, and Zelrix)

**Table 1**
Acute therapies for migraine

| Group 1[a] | Group 2[b] | Group 3[c] | Group 4[d] | Group 5[e] |
|---|---|---|---|---|
| Specific | Acetaminophen plus codeine PO | Butalbital, aspirin, plus caffeine PO | Acetaminophen PO | Dexamethasone IV |
| Naratriptan PO | Butalbital, aspirin, caffeine, plus codeine PO | Ergotamine PO | Chlorpromazine IM | Hydrocortisone IV |
| Rizatriptan PO | Butorphanol IM | Ergotamine plus caffeine PO | Granisetron IV | |
| Sumatriptan SC, IN, PO | Chlorpromazine IM, IV | Metoclopramide IM, PR | Lidocaine IV | |
| Zolmitriptan PO | Diclofenac K, PO | | | |
| DHE SC, IM, IV, IN | Ergotamine plus caffeine plus pentobarbital plus Bellafoline PO | | | |
| DHE IV, plus antiemetic | Flurbiprofen, PO | | | |
| Nonspecific | Isometheptere CPD, PO | | | |
| Acetaminophen, aspirin, plus caffeine PO | Ketorolac IM | | | |
| Aspirin PO | Lidocaine IN | | | |
| Butorphanol IN | Meperidine IM, IV | | | |
| Ibuprofen PO | Methadone IM | | | |
| Naproxen sodium PO | Metoclopram de IV | | | |
| Prochlorperazine IV | Naproxen PO Prochlorperazine IM, PR | | | |

*Abbreviations:* IM, intramuscularly; IV, intravenously; PO, orally; PR, per rectum; SC, subcutaneously.
[a] Proven, pronounced statistical and clinical benefit (≥2 double-blind, placebo-controlled studies and clinical impression of effect).
[b] Moderate statistical and clinical benefit (1 double-blind, placebo-controlled study and clinical impression of effect).
[c] Statistically but not proven clinically or clinically but not proven statistically effective (conflicting or inconsistent evidence).
[d] Proven to be statistically or clinically ineffective (failed efficacy vs placebo).
[e] Clinical and statistical benefits unknown (insufficient evidence available).

*From* Silberstein SD. Practice parameter: evidence-based guidelines for migraine headache (an evidence-based review): report of the quality standards subcommittee of the American academy of neurology. Neurology 2000;55(6):754–62; with permission.

has been used for treatment, as well as parenteral dihydroergotamine (given intramuscularly, subcutaneously, intravenously, or intranasally). The recommended doses are as follows[11,12]:

- Imitrex injection: 6 mg subcutaneously; may repeat if needed more than 1 hour after initial dose (maximum of two 6-mg injections in a 24-hour period).
- Imitrex nasal: 5 mg in 1 nostril; or 10 mg (5 mg in each nostril); or 20 mg. May repeat the dose in 2 hours if the headache returns. The dosage should not exceed 40 mg in 24 hours.
- Sumatriptan transdermal (Zelrix): One patch (6.5 mg) for 4 hours. May apply a second patch after the first patch has been on for no less than 2 hours. The patient may apply a maximum of 2 patches in a 24-hour period.
- Migranal IM or subcutaneous: 1 mg at first sign of migraine headache. The dose may be repeated every hour to a maximum dosage of 3 mg/d and 6 mg/wk.
- Migranal IV: 1 mg at first sign of migraine headache. The dose may be repeated hourly to a maximum dosage of 2 mg/d and 6 mg/wk.
- Migranal intranasal: 1 spray (0.5 mg) in each nostril at first sign of migraine headache. The dose may be repeated after 15 minutes to a maximum of 4 sprays (2 mg). The patient should not exceed 6 sprays (2 mg) in a 24-hour period and no more than 8 sprays (4 mg) in a week.

## PEDIATRICS

The treatment of migraine headache in children is very similar to treatment in adults. The suggested initial treatment is the use of a simple analgesic.[13] The analgesics of choice are acetaminophen (Tylenol) or ibuprofen (Motrin, Advil). The doses are as follows:

- Ibuprofen (Motrin, Advil): 10 mg/kg at the onset of migraine headache. The dose may be repeated in 4 to 6 hours but should not exceed 4 doses in 24 hours (maximum of 40 mg/kg).
- Acetaminophen (Tylenol): 10 to 20 mg/kg (maximum of 1000 mg) at the onset of migraine headache. The dose may be repeated in 2 to 4 hours and the patient may not take more than 3 doses in 24 hours.

Children who have mild to moderate migraine headaches with nausea and vomiting should be given an antiemetic. The antiemetic of choice is promethazine (Phenergan) 0.25 to 0.5 mg/kg per rectum. The dosage may be repeated every 4 to 6 hours as needed.

Children who have migraine headaches without vomiting but do not respond to simple analgesics are treated with oral triptans. Sumatriptan (Imitrex oral) is the triptan of choice. The starting dose of oral sumatriptan is 25 mg (maximum dose of 50 mg). However, children who are unable to take sumatriptan may take either rizatriptan (Maxalt) 5 mg wafer, zolmitriptan (Zomig) 2.5 or 5 mg, or almotriptan (Axert) 6.25 or 12.5 mg. Rizatriptan and zolmitriptan are preferred for children with early nausea and vomiting because they are available in orally disintegrating formulations.

A combination of oral sumatriptan-naproxen is recommended for children with migraine and no vomiting who do not respond to monotherapy with other medications. A randomized, parallel group of 12 to 17 year olds was studied to determine with pain free rates from baseline after 2 hours.[2] Sumatriptan-naproxen doses of 10/60 mg, 30/180 mg, and 85/500 mg were studied with significant differences found at the 85/500 mg dose versus placebo (23% vs 9%; $P = .008$).

Children who are at least 5 years old and do not respond to analgesics, have persistent vomiting, and cannot take the orally disintegrating formulations should use sumatriptan (Imitrex) nasal spray, starting with a 5-mg dose. The dose can be repeated once in 4 to 6 hours if the child initially felt relief from the migraine headache but the headache returned. Children who felt no relief should try the 10 mg nasal spray (two 5-mg sprays given together). The nasal spray may be used at a higher dosage (maximum of 20 mg) in older children. Children are asked to suck a hard piece of candy after using the nasal spray because the spray leaves a bad taste in the mouth. Zolmitriptan (Zomig) nasal spray (5 mg) may be used if the child does not like or want to use sumatriptan nasal spray.[13]

## NONPHARMACOLOGIC TREATMENT OPTIONS

The American Academy of Neurology (AAN) made recommendations in 2000 for non-pharmacologic treatment of migraine.[14] The AAN recommended relaxation training, thermal biofeedback combined with relaxation training, electromyographic biofeed-back, and cognitive–behavioral therapy, but the AAN was unable to state what type of patient would benefit best from these therapies. The AAN also suggested that behavioral therapy would work well with preventative drug therapy. The AAN could not make recommendations for the use of hypnosis, acupuncture, transcutaneous electrical nerve stimulation, chiropractic or osteopathic cervical manipulation, occlusal adjustment (adjusting patient's bite), or hyperbaric oxygen.

## SURGICAL TREATMENT OPTIONS

Patients who have been unable to find relief with pharmacologic and nonpharmacologic options can seek out surgical treatment. One surgery involves the removal of trigger sites for headache.[15] The surgical deactivation of migraine trigger sites has been found to be an effective treatment for patients who have frequent moderate to severe migraine headaches. Another option that has been recommended in the past was closure of the patent foramen ovale. However, a retrospective analysis of the procedure showed low availability of evidence to conclude that the surgery is effective.[16]

## MIGRAINE VARIANTS

Migraine variants include hemiplegic migraine (either familial or sporadic), menstrual migraine, basilar-type migraine, and retinal migraine. Hemiplegic migraine is charac-terized by motor weakness on 1 side of the body during a migraine attack. Basilar type migraine is associated with blurred vision, syncope, and ataxia. Menstrual migraine occurs 2 days before to 3 days after the beginning of a menstrual cycle. Retinal migraine is characterized by visual disturbances or blindness for up to 1 hour (**Table 2**).[3]

**Table 2**
**Migraine variants**

| Migraine Variant | Onset | Characterization |
| --- | --- | --- |
| Basilar | During migraine | Blurred vision, syncope, ataxia |
| Hemiplegic | During migraine | Motor weakness on one side of the body |
| Menstrual | Two days before to 3 d after beginning of menstrual cycle | Typical migraine |
| Retinal | During migraine | Visual disturbances of blindness for $\leq 1$ h |

**Table 3**
**Treatment of migraines**

| Age Group | Severity of Migraine | Medication | Recommended Start Time |
|-----------|---------------------|------------|------------------------|
| Adult (>18 y old) | Mild to moderate | NSAIDs (aspirin, ibuprofen, naproxen, etc) Treximet | Onset of migraine |
| | Mild to moderate with nausea and vomiting | NSAID or Treximet plus Metoclopramide | Onset of migraine |
| | Moderate to Severe | Triptans (Eletriptan, Naratriptan, etc) | Onset of migraine |
| | Moderate to severe with nausea and vomiting | Parenteral (Imitrex injection, Imitrex nasal, Zelrix, Migranal, etc) | Onset of migraine |
| Children | Mild to moderate | NSAIDs (Acetaminophen or Ibuprofen) | Onset of migraine |
| | Mild to moderate with nausea and vomiting | NSAIDs plus Promethazine | Onset of migraine |
| | Mild to moderate unresponsive to simple analgesics | Triptans (sumatriptan preferred) | Onset of migraine |
| | Mild to moderate with no vomiting and unresponsive to monotherapy | Combination Sumatriptan-Naproxen | Onset of migraine |
| | At least 5 y old and unresponsive to analgesics with persistent vomiting and unable to take orally disintegrating formulations | Sumatriptan nasal spray | Onset of migraine |

*Abbreviation:* NSAIDs, nonsteroidal anti-inflammatory drugs.

## SUMMARY

The acute treatment of migraine should start early with an effective dose. Children and adults should start with simple analgesics for mild to moderate migraine headaches without vomiting. Those children and adults who do not respond to monotherapy can try sumatriptan–naproxen (Treximet) as a treatment strategy. Adults with mild to moderate migraine headache and vomiting should add an antiemetic to their regimen. Metoclopramide is recommended for adult patients; promethazine is recommended for children. Finally, children and adults with moderate to severe migraine should try parenteral therapies like sumatriptan nasal spray (**Table 3**). Relaxation training and cognitive behavioral therapy have a role in nonpharmacologic treatment options and surgical removal of trigger points has been found to be effective.[15]

## REFERENCES

1. Charles A. The evolution of a migraine attack- a review of recent evidence. Headache 2013;53(2):413.
2. Silberstein SD. Practice parameter: evidence-based guidelines for migraine headache (an evidence-based review): report of the quality standards subcommittee of the American Academy of Neurology. Neurology 2000;55(6):754–62.

3. Headache Classification Committee of the International Headache Society (HIS). The international classification of headache disorders, 3rd edition (beta version). Cephalalgia 2013;33(9):629–808.
4. Stafstrom CE, Rostasy K, Minster A. The usefulness of children's drawings in the diagnosis of headache. Pediatrics 2002;109(3):460.
5. Trottier ED, Bailey B, Lucas N, et al. Diagnosis of migraine in the pediatric emergency department. Pediatr Neurol 2013;49(1):40–5.
6. Lipton RB, Stewart WF, Stone AM, et al. Stratified care vs. step care strategies for migraine: the disability in strategies of care (DISC) study; a randomized trial. JAMA 2000;284(20):2599.
7. UpToDate. Acute treatment of migraine in adults. 2014. Available at: http://www.uptodate.com/contents/acute-treatment-of-migraine-in-adults?source=search_result&search=acute+treatment+of+migraine&selectedTitle=1%7E150. Accessed March 24, 2014.
8. Brandes JL, Kudrow D, Start SR, et al. Sumatriptan-naproxen for acute treatment of migraine; a randomized trial. JAMA 2007;297(13):1443.
9. Tfelt-Hansen P, Henry P, Mulder LJ, et al. The effectiveness of combined oral lysine acetysalicylate and metoclopramide compared with oral sumatriptan for migraine. Lancet 1995;346(8980):923.
10. UpToDate. Sumatriptan: drug information lexicomp. Available at: http://www.uptodate.com/contents/sumatriptan-drug-information?source=see_link&utdPopup=true. Accessed March 26, 2014.
11. UpToDate. Dihydroergotamine: drug information lexicomp. Available at: http://www.uptodate.com/contents/dihydroergotamine-drug-information?source=see_link&utdPopup=true. Accessed March 26, 2014.
12. UpToDate. Management of migraine headache in children. 2014. Available at: http://www.uptodate.com/contents/management-of-migraine-headache-in-children?source=search_result&search=migraine+in+children&selectedTitle=2%7E150#H29. Accessed March 27, 2014.
13. Derosier FJ, Lewis D, Hershey AD, et al. Randomized trial of sumatriptan and naproxen sodium combination in adolescent migraine. Pediatrics 2013;129(6):e1411.
14. Guyuron B, Reed D, Kriegler JS, et al. A placebo-controlled surgical trial of the treatment of migraine headaches. Plast Reconstr Surg 2009;124(2):461.
15. Schwedt TJ, Demaerschalk BM, Dodick DW. Patent foramen ovale and migraine; a quantitative systematic review. Cephalalgia 2008;28(5):531.
16. UpToDate. Preventive treatment of migraine in adults. 2014. Available at: http://www.uptodate.com/contents/preventive-treatment-of-migraine-in-adults?source=search_result&search=migraine+prevention&selectedTitle=1%7E150. Accessed March 31, 2014.

# Sports-Related Traumatic Brain Injury

Shawn Phillips, MD[a], Derek Woessner, MD[b],*

## KEYWORDS

- Sports-related • Mild traumatic brain injury • MTBI • Mild TBI guidelines
- Sideline Concussion Assessment Tool 3 (SCAT3) • Postconcussive syndrome

## KEY POINTS

- The term *concussion* has been supplanted by the term *mild traumatic brain injury* (MTBI), but the two are still used interchangeably.
- The definition for MTBI is a "complex pathophysiologic process affecting the brain, induced by traumatic biomechanical forces secondary to direct or indirect forces to the head."
- SCAT3 is common sideline assessment tool.
- Any one symptom or sign of concussion should prompt removal of the athlete from play for the remainder of the event.
- Neuroimaging is rarely necessary for the diagnosis of concussion.

## INTRODUCTION

In his work on the gladiator games of the Roman Empire, Galen (129–216/217 AD) documented sports-related traumatic brain injuries (TBI).[1] In the present day, concussions have garnered more attention in the medical literature, media, and social media. Therefore, in the nomenclature according to the Centers for Disease Control and Prevention, "Facts for Physicians" the term *concussion* has been supplanted by the term *mild TBI* (MTBI).[2] And MTBI is defined as a "complex pathophysiologic process affecting the brain, induced by traumatic biomechanical forces secondary to direct or indirect forces to the head." Current numbers indicate that 1.7 million are documented TBIs annually, with estimates around 3 million annually (173,285 sports- and recreation-related TBIs among children and adolescents). The Sideline Concussion Assessment Tool 3 (SCAT3) and the NFL Sideline Concussion Assessment Tool are commonly used sideline tools.

---

The authors have nothing to disclose.
[a] 555 North Duke Street, Lancaster, PA 17602, USA; [b] Lancaster General Hospital, 555 North Duke Street, Lancaster, PA 17602, USA
* Corresponding author.
*E-mail address:* dwoessner2@lghealth.org

## MANAGEMENT GOALS

Management of concussion in sport consists of several phases:

- Evaluation of airway, breathing, and cardiovascular function
- Evaluation of the cervical spine
  - Immobilization and transfer to an appropriate trauma center is necessary if cervical spine injury is suspected
- Evaluation for signs of rapidly worsening mental status
  - Focal neurologic findings, including abnormal pupillary response, abnormal extraocular movements, and abnormal motor or sensory functions should be ruled out
  - Immediate transfer to an appropriate trauma center with neuroimaging capabilities is indicated for any signs of neurologic deterioration

Neuroimaging is rarely necessary for the diagnosis of MTBI.[3,4] It should be considered to rule out any more serious brain injury or skull fracture. Computed tomography can be used in an acute setting when focal symptoms are noted to rule out mass effect. It is also the best tool when skull fracture is considered. MRI may also be considered in the evaluation of persistent symptoms that do not resolve as expected.

See **Box 1** for goals of concussion management.

## SIDELINE MANAGEMENT

After serious cervical spine or brain injury is ruled out, further evaluation can commence. All athletes with suspected brain injury should be removed from competition until evaluated by a licensed health care provider with experience in the evaluation of MTBIs.[3,4] Current guidelines recommend the use of a standardized sideline tool in evaluating an athlete with a suspected MTBI.[3] Several sideline tools are available for the management of MTBI. The most commonly used tools currently available combine health history with testing of cognition and assessment of balance. Balance testing most commonly used is based on the Balance Error Scoring System (BESS). BESS is a 5-minute test using 3 standing positions (double leg stance, single leg stance, and tandem stance) to evaluate balance on multiple surfaces.[3] The BESS is 34% sensitive and 94% specific in predicting concussion.[3]

Current sideline tools use Modified BESS testing, which tests same standing positions but on a firm surface only - no studies have shown its sensitivity or specificity.[3,5] The Sideline Concussion Assessment Tool 3 (SCAT3) and the NFL Sideline Concussion Assessment Tool are commonly used sideline tools.[3,6] The SCAT3 was recently updated from the SCAT2 to include questions about relevant history, including history of migraine headache, attention-deficit/hyperactivity disorder, depression, and anxiety and an inquiry about current medications.[3] The SCAT3 is normed for all individuals

---

**Box 1**
**Concussion management goals**

Initial evaluation and diagnosis

Postinjury evaluation

Symptom management

Safe return to participation

aged 13 years and older. The Child-SCAT3 test is available to evaluate children aged 12 years and younger.

Any one symptom or sign of MTBI should prompt removal of the athlete from play for the remainder of the event (**Boxes 2** and **3**).[3,5] Athletes diagnosed with MTBI should not be left unattended and should be reevaluated on the sideline periodically to monitor for any signs of deteriorating neurologic status. Any signs of deterioration should prompt transfer to an appropriate emergency department for further evaluation.

An athlete with MTBI, if a minor, should be accompanied home by a parent/guardian, or, if an adult, by a responsible caregiver. These caregivers should be educated about signs and symptoms of worsening neurologic status, but do not need to wake the individual with concussion from sleep to reevaluate. In the days following an MTBI, the athlete will need to be evaluated for the persistence of symptoms and to determine when safe return to participation can be allowed.

## INTERVENTIONS
### Pharmacologic Strategies

Few pharmacologic interventions have been shown to be beneficial in the initial management of an MTBI. Management focuses on individual symptoms. Headache in the days following concussion can be treated with nonsteroidal anti-inflammatory drugs (NSAIDs) or acetaminophen and rest. Headache that persists may require further treatment. Abortive therapies beyond NSAIDs or acetaminophen for a migraine or tension-type headache can be considered and used as indicated.[3,4] Headache associated with an MTBI can persist for weeks or beyond when associated with postconcussion syndrome. Management of persistent headache may require prophylactic medications. Options for prophylactic medications for concussion commonly include nonspecific ß-blockers and tricyclic antidepressants, although little evidence supports the use of any particular prophylactic medication for headache after concussion. Persistent headache after concussion should be managed as part of a comprehensive management plan for postconcussive syndrome.[3,7] Balance disturbance secondary to vertigo is common in the days following an MTBI. Benzodiazepines and meclizine can be used for symptom control. Balance difficulties that persist because of postconcussive syndrome should be managed as part of a comprehensive strategy.

### Nonpharmacologic Strategies

For many Individuals with an MTBI, symptoms resolve after a few days of cognitive and physical rest. The average time for resolution of symptoms is 7 to

| Box 2 |
| --- |
| **Symptoms of concussion** |
| Headache |
| Dizziness |
| Lightheadedness |
| Vision changes |
| Drowsiness |
| Nausea/vomiting |

| Box 3 |
| --- |
| **Physical signs of concussion** |
| Impaired concentration |
| Irritability |
| Anxiety |
| Impaired memory |
| Impaired balance testing |
| Impaired coordination |

10 days.[3,4,6–8] Currently, treatment focuses mainly on the management of symptoms. Sleep disturbances are common, but in the days following an MTBI, these should not require medications to manage. No evidence supports medications to promote sleep in the first several days after concussion.[3] The focus should be on good sleep hygiene.

Alterations of mood, such as anxiety and depression, are common. No evidence supports the use of medications in the first several weeks after concussion to address condition-related mood disturbances. Symptoms that persist beyond 6 weeks may require further evaluation. Athletes with baseline mood issues will need to be monitored closely after MTBI for any acute changes, and these should be managed appropriately.

Decreased attention is a common symptom in the days following an MTBI,[3] although no evidence supports the use of stimulant medication to manage MTBI-related attention deficits. Athletes with baseline attention-deficit disorder should continue with their prescribed treatments.

### Self-Management Strategies

In the days after concussion, the goal of symptom management is cognitive and physical rest. Initially, athletes should avoid activities that can worsen symptoms. Cognitive rest includes avoidance of activities that require ocular focus, such as reading, watching TV, and using a computer or other electronic devices. Avoidance of all physical activity that worsens symptoms is also recommended in the days after concussion. Symptom management can include resting in a dark, quiet environment to avoid exacerbation of headache.

### REEVALUATION

MTBI requires regular reevaluation in the days to weeks after the initial injury. The average time from injury to return to participation is 7 to 10 days. Cognitive and physical rest is the mainstay of MTBI management in the days after concussion. Computerized neuropsychological testing can be considered before return to play once an individual is without symptoms.[3,9] This is an objective test to measure brain behavior.

Computerized testing has some moderate evidence to detect postconcussive cognitive dysfunction that exists beyond the time a concussed individual is symptomatic. Baseline testing may be helpful in evaluating an individual's postconcussion deficits. No specific evidence-based recommendations currently exist for postconcussion neuropsychological testing. Computerized neuropsychological testing should only be used as an adjunct to the comprehensive management of concussion.

| Box 4 |
| Stage of recovery |
| --- |
| No activity |
| Light aerobics |
| Sport-specific training |
| Noncontact drills |
| Full contact participation |
| Return to participation |

## RETURN TO PARTICIPATION

Return to play is permitted once an individual is asymptomatic. Return to play is a stepwise, gradual program in which the last step is full participation in the preinjury activity. Evidence supports a graduated return-to-play protocol, such as depicted in **Box 4**.[3] Symptoms at any stage of recovery should prompt halting of the protocol progression and a return to the previous stage.[3,10,11] Return to play should be supervised by a qualified health professional familiar with the management of concussion.[3,10,11]

## POSTCONCUSSIVE SYNDROME

Postconcussive syndrome is the presence of symptoms of concussion that persist for several weeks after injury. Most concussions resolve within 7 to 10 days. The cause of postconcussive syndrome is unknown. Risk factors for postconcussive syndrome are female sex, increasing age, and non–sports-related concussion.[3,7] Management of postconcussive syndrome consists of time and patience. Modified activity at work or school may be required. Postconcussive syndrome should be managed by an interdisciplinary team.[3,7]

## RECURRENCE

Some evidence indicates that chronic cognitive issues may be associated with recurrent concussion.[12] Prolonged symptoms seem to be present in patients with more than 2 to 3 lifetime concussions. More studies are needed for evaluation.[5,7,8,12]

## SUMMARY

The topic of concussions and MTBIs in sports has gained increased media attention and a renewed focus in the medical community. Medical providers are key in the prevention of MTBIs and their early identification, management, and treatment. Guidelines, such as SCAT3, can improve patient outcomes by allowing providers to more readily diagnose an MTBI and refer patients when needed. Additionally, providers should recognize that MTBIs are not limited to collision sports such as football, but span the continuum to include contact sports (eg, soccer) and noncontact sports (eg, cheerleading). Any one symptom or sign of concussion should prompt removal of the athlete from play for the remainder of the event. In the days following a concussion, the athlete should be evaluated to determine persistence of symptoms. Return to play is a stepwise, gradual program in which the last step is full participation in the preinjury activity. Evidence supports a graduated return to play protocol. Symptoms at any stage of recovery should prompt halting of the protocol progression and a return to the previous stage.

## REFERENCES

1. Wrightson P. The development of a concept of mild head injury. J Clin Neurosci 2000;7:384–8.
2. Centers for Disease Control and Prevention, National Center for Injury Prevention and Control. Facts for physicians. In: Heads up: brain injury in your practice. Atlanta (GA): Center for Disease Control and Prevention; 2007. p. 2. Available at: http://www.cdc.gov/ncipc/tbi/Physicians Tool Kit.htm.
3. Harmon KG, Drezner JA, Gammons M, et al. American Medical Society for Sports Medicine position statement: concussion in sport. Br J Sports Med 2013;47: 15–26.
4. Gravel J, D'Angelo A, Carrière B, et al. Interventions provided in the acute phase for mild traumatic brain injury: a systematic review. Syst Rev 2013;2:63.
5. Christman SP, Schiff MA, Chung SK, et al. Implementation of concussion legislation and extent of concussion education for athletes, parents and coaches in Washington state. Am J Sports Med 2014;42(5):1190–6.
6. Guskiewicz KM. Balance assessment in the management of sport-related concussion. Clin Sports Med 2011;30:63–72.
7. Ryan LM, Warden DL. Post concussion syndrome. Int Rev Psychiatry 2003;15: 310–6.
8. Cantu RC. Recurrent athletic head injury; risks and when to retire. Clin Sports Med 2003;22:593–603.
9. Randolph C. Baseline neuropsychological testing in managing sport-related concussion: doesit modify risk? Curr Sports Med Rep 2011;10:21–6.
10. Rivara FP, Schiff MA, Chrisman SP, et al. The effect of coach education on reporting of concussions among high school athletes after passage of a concussion law. Am J Sports Med 2014;42(5):1197–203.
11. Shrey DW, Griesbach GS, Giza CC. The pathophysiology of concussions in youth. Phys Med Rehabil Clin N Am 2011;22:577–602, vii.
12. Sedney CL, Orphanos J, Biles JE. When to consider retiring an athlete after sports-related concussion. Clin Sports Med 2011;30:189–200.

# Office Evaluation of Dizziness

James D. Hogue, DO

## KEYWORDS

- Dizziness • Vertigo • Presyncope • Syncope • Disequilibrium
- Nonspecific dizziness • Dix-Hallpike maneuver • Nystagmus

## KEY POINTS

- Patients presenting to primary care with complaints of dizziness are common.
- Differentiating the cause of dizziness can be made easier by considering 4 main categories of dizziness: vertigo, presyncope/syncope, disequilibrium, and nonspecific symptoms.
- Differentials should immediately include the most common causes of dizziness, such as benign paroxysmal positional vertigo and orthostatic hypotension.
- Diagnostic tests should be ordered for patients who have abnormal findings on physical examination that may indicate a more serious cause of dizziness.

## INTRODUCTION

Dizziness is a common concern in primary care practice. Dizziness will affect 20% to 30% of the general population of patients seen in a primary care setting.[1–4] Patients' complaints of dizziness can be both challenging and time-consuming because of the vagueness and ambiguity of the symptoms and the wide variety of possible diagnoses.[5,6] As a complaint, "dizziness" is a nonspecific term used by patients to describe a wide variety of symptoms. Differentiating the type of dizziness can be difficult but is essential in the course of an evaluation.[7] It is most helpful to try to categorize dizziness into one of the following groups:

- Vertigo
- Presyncope/syncope
- Disequilibrium
- Non-specific

Peripheral vestibular disease, vertigo, is the most common diagnosis in dizzy patients.[5,8,9] The most common of the peripheral vestibular disorders is benign

Georgia Campus, Philadelphia College of Osteopathic Medicine, 625 Old Peachtree Road NW, Suwanee, GA 30024, USA
E-mail address: jdhogue@charter.net

Prim Care Clin Office Pract 42 (2015) 249–258
http://dx.doi.org/10.1016/j.pop.2015.01.004
0095-4543/15/$ – see front matter © 2015 Elsevier Inc. All rights reserved.

paroxysmal positional vertigo (BPPV) followed by Meniere disease and vestibular neuritis (labyrinthitis).[5,6,8,9] The second most common disorder is orthostatic hypotension.[5] Multiple sensory deficits are common in the elderly and lead to problems with disequilibrium that are often described as "dizziness."

Brain tumors are rare findings in patients with dizziness.[1,10] Fewer than 10% of patients complaining of dizziness have been affected by serious cardiac or neurologic disorders such as arrhythmias or stroke.[5] By categorizing the symptoms and physical findings, a diagnosis for the cause of the dizziness can be made more than 80% of the time.[5] The first important step is to fit the patient into one of the categories. The next section describes the pathophysiology of each category.

## PATHOPHYSIOLOGY
### Vertigo

Vertigo occurs when there is an asymmetry in the vestibular system.[11] This asymmetry causes an illusion of motion that can be described as self-motion or motion of the environment. The most common description is a "spinning sensation." The illusion of motion is usually brought on by and exaggerated by head movement.[11] The vestibular system pathway controls balance and eye movements. Impairment of the pathway causes a sensory overload leading the brain to misinterpret the data. Peripheral vertigo (most common) is usually caused by a disturbance in the inner ear that affects the labyrinth or the vestibular nerve, such as BPPV, Meniere disease, and labyrinthitis. Central vertigo (uncommon) is usually caused by an underlying medical disorder, such as cerebrovascular disease, brain stem lesions, stroke, multiple sclerosis, possible tumors, and migraine headaches.[7,12–15] BPPV (the most common peripheral cause) is caused by displaced otoliths from the utricle and saccule. The displaced otoliths tend to settle in the most dependent portion of the ear, the posterior semicircular canal, and occasionally in the lateral semicircular canal. Movement of the otoliths in the canal cause exaggerated movement of the endolymph, creating an imbalance in the signal resulting in vertigo. Meniere disease is poorly understood in terms of the cause and pathophysiology.[5,16] A common finding is dilated endolymph channels thought to be caused by an obstruction that results in increased endolymph pressure that creates breaks in the intralabyrinthine membranes, resulting in vertigo, tinnitus, and hearing loss.[5,16–18] Vestibular neuritis is more commonly known as labyrinthitis. The problem is thought to be virally mediated causing a mononeuropathy of the vestibular division of the eighth cranial nerve on one side. Many patients complain of a preceding viral illness. There is also evidence that some cases of labyrinthitis are caused by reactivation of latent herpes simplex virus type 1 infection.[5,19] Migraine headaches causing a sensation of vertigo are fairly common.

### Presyncope/Syncope

Presyncope is described as a near faint or the prodromal symptom of fainting,[11] which typically results from cerebral hypoperfusion or cardiac irregularities.[7] Patients with cardiovascular disease are at risk for orthostatic hypotension and cardiac arrhythmias.[1,20] Orthostatic hypotension has been found to be the second most common cause of complaints of dizziness.[5] Dizziness during the act of standing can point to symptoms associated with orthostatic hypotension when the cardiovascular system cannot react appropriately to gravitational changes that occur when going from supine to standing erect. Cardiac rate-controlling medications may blunt the necessary heart rate response when standing up, leading to orthostatic hypotension. Diuretic medications may lead to degrees of hypovolemia, a common cause of orthostatic hypotension.[7] Vasovagal reactions with the resulting sudden decrease in blood pressure can be considered in this category.[11] Whenever there is concern that a cardiovascular problem is the cause of dizziness, a full cardiac examination should be performed with consideration given to an evaluation by a cardiologist.

## Disequilibrium

Disequilibrium is a sense of imbalance primarily when walking. Chronic disequilibrium can cause significant impairment of physical and social functioning, particularly in the elderly.[11,21,22] Musculoskeletal disorders, peripheral neuropathy, vestibular disorders, cerebellar disorders, and cervical spondylosis may result in disequilibrium.[11,23,24] Visual impairment usually exacerbates the sense of imbalance.[11] A disturbance in postural control secondary to cervical spondylosis often causes dizziness. Patients with Parkinson disease can suffer from postural hypotension as well as a significant sense of imbalance.[11,25] Involvement of the cerebellar hemisphere causes incoordination of the limbs, thereby having a significant effect on gait. Cerebrovascular accident and transient ischemic attack (TIA) (vertebrobasilar insufficiency) can cause staggering when walking, feelings of imbalance (disequilibrium), and a falling sensation.[1] Patients with central causes of dizziness and disequilibrium are often unable to stand or ambulate without assistance.[1] Unsteadiness related to postural control is mostly a result of neurologic disorders that do not exhibit vestibular impairment.[7,15] The most common cause of disequilibrium is multiple sensory deficits.[7,26,27] The accumulation of multiple sensory insults deprives patients of enough sensory information about the environment to cause the presenting complaint to be dizziness.[5,28]

## Nonspecific Dizziness

In general, a categorization of nonspecific dizziness results when the patient has difficulty describing their symptoms. Patients may incorporate symptoms common to all of the other categories, making differentiation difficult. Symptoms described as dizziness in psychiatric disorders often have to be placed in this nonspecific category.[11] One of the most common causes of nonspecific dizziness is hyperventilation. Hypoglycemic episodes often cause nonspecific dizziness.[11,29] Medications, especially antidepressants and anticholinergics, produce side effects, causing nonspecific dizziness with the symptoms becoming worse with abrupt drug withdrawal.[11,30,31] Most patients with nonspecific dizziness are healthy, young individuals that show no evidence of disease involving the neurologic, cardiovascular, or otolaryngologic systems. Psychological disturbances, such as anxiety, panic attacks, depression, or the medications used to treat these disorders, may result in dizziness. Nonspecific dizziness is not clearly defined and is not related to positional changes or orthostatic hypotension.[7,32,33]

## HISTORY

Some studies have shown that the history has proven to be the most sensitive means for establishing a category for dizzy complaints.[11,34] History alone can reveal the diagnosis in approximately 75% of patients complaining of dizziness.[1,10] A thorough general history followed by a focused history can allow the patient to provide a description that is critical for establishing the cause of the dizziness.[11,34] Asking open-ended questions allows the patient to describe his or her symptoms. Then, checking and gathering additional information from focused, specific questions should help establish a category.[11] It is important to place the symptoms into context, including time, course, aggravating and relieving factors, concurrent symptoms, age, and pre-existing conditions.[7]

## Typical History by Category

### Vertigo

All vertigo is made worse by moving the head. Patients with vertigo are frequently afraid to move.[11] Vertigo is abrupt in onset, episodic, and always aggravated by head movements.[5,6,23] Patients state that they are spinning or the room is spinning. Other frequent descriptions are rotating, twirling, or swaying. Lack of spinning cannot be used to exclude vestibular disease. True vertigo is never continuous for more than a few weeks. The central nervous system adapts to the defect and the vertigo subsides over the course of several weeks.[11] It is important to be clear on what is meant by "constant" dizziness. Some patients may have a constant susceptibility to frequent, episodic dizziness that is actually a vestibular problem. Vertigo is often accompanied by nausea, vomiting, diaphoresis, and blurry vision.[11] Severe nausea and vomiting are more common with peripheral than central lesions.[7,14,35] Symptoms of dizziness from vertigo and presyncope can often be confused because both are associated with dizziness on standing. The key to determination is doing maneuvers that change head position without lowering blood pressure.[11] Ear symptoms with vertigo can include tinnitus, pain or pressure, and changes in hearing. Meniere disease may cause a more sustained vertigo that is more disabling and more severe than vertigo from BPPV. An associated complaint may be fluctuating hearing loss.[1,10,36] Migraine-associated vertigo goes along with typical migraine symptoms. Photophobia, phono-phobia, and auras are common along with vertigo. Duration may last from 5 minutes to an hour.[1,37] Past head trauma is a common cause of BPPV. Patients may also report an upper respiratory illness just before the onset of symptoms. Vertigo of central origin impairs gait and posture to a greater degree than peripheral vertigo. Patients with peripheral vertigo are usually able to walk but may be reluctant to do so.[11] Recurrent vertigo lasting less than a minute is usually BPPV.[11,38] Single episodes lasting several minutes to hours may be migraine related or indicate a TIA.[6,11] Recurrent episodes associated with Meniere disease typically last for hours.[11,39,40] More prolonged, severe episodes that occur with vestibular neuritis can last for days.[4,11]

### Presyncope/syncope

Presyncope is a state of lightheadedness or a feeling of imminent loss of conscious-ness.[7,12] Syncope occurs with a transient loss of consciousness or a "blackout."[7,41,42] The transient "blackout" can be accompanied by visual changes (graying of vision) and a lack of awareness of the surroundings.[7,43] The history will reveal that the symp-toms are worse with standing and are relieved by laying down.[7,44] Complaints such as palpitations, shortness of breath, and chest pain should point to a cardiac cause of the symptoms. Patients with histories of cardiovascular disease may be at risk for cardiac arrhythmias and may be affected by heart rate–controlling and diuretic medications.

### Disequilibrium

Disequilibrium is usually characterized by complaints of shakiness or a sense of imbal-ance while walking.[7] The symptoms may be reported as dizziness when, in fact, they are just unsteady on their feet. The sense of imbalance with disequilibrium worsens with darkness and can change the length and width of the patient's steps.[7,26,45] Patients will report the use of a cane or using furniture for contact guarding during ambula-tion.[7,15] Disequilibrium is a sensation of unsteadiness not related to head movement, implying that it is a proprioceptive problem or possibly cerebellar disease.[5,6,23]

## Nonspecific

Symptoms that do not reasonably fit the other categories are then considered nonspecific. It is important to consider central lesions when the symptoms appear to be classified to this category. Complaints of dizziness associated with anxiety or depression should prompt an evaluation for psychological causes.[7,10,46] It is important to obtain a medication history, including over-the-counter medications, many of which can cause dizziness as a side effect. Consideration should also be given to a history of nontraditional or alternative medications and therapies.[7] Symptoms associated with vertebrobasilar insufficiency include a sudden onset of vertigo that can last for days without improvement. Associated symptoms would include ataxia, dysphagia, confusion, double vision or visual loss, slurred speech, and numbness.[7,27,33] Any symptoms that point to central causes of dizziness warrant immediate further investigation.[7] Patients with central causes of dizziness and vertigo are often unable to stand or ambulate without assistance. Patients with an episode of dizziness and one or more stroke risk factors have a substantial risk of subsequent stroke.[2,47] Certain medications are associated with vestibular dysfunction (aminoglycosides) or cerebellar toxicity (phenytoin). Dizziness in older patients that is difficult to categorize has been found to be independently associated with 7 characteristics[11]:

- Anxiety trait
- Depressive symptoms
- Impaired balance
- Post myocardial infarction
- Postural hypotension
- Five or more medications
- Impaired hearing

## PHYSICAL EXAMINATION

A thorough physical examination and a focused neurologic examination are essential for evaluating complaints of dizziness. The physical examination characteristics typically found for each category follow.

### Vertigo

Vertigo, whether central or peripheral in origin, is generally accompanied by nystagmus and postural instability. The presence of nystagmus suggests that the dizziness is vertigo. The bilateral symmetric appearance of a few beats of horizontal nystagmus on lateral gaze is normal (physiologic "endpoint" nystagmus). Pathologic nystagmus is asymmetric or more pronounced or prolonged.[11] The presence of additional neurologic signs strongly suggests the presence of a central vestibular lesion. Staggering gait or ataxic gait, vomiting, headache, double vision, visual loss, slurred speech, numbness of the face or body, weakness, clumsiness, or incoordination should prompt an evaluation for a central lesion. It is common though for patients with true vertigo (nystagmus present) to have difficulty maintaining a steady upright posture when walking, standing, or even sitting unsupported.[11] Nystagmus is a rhythmic oscillation of the eyes. In a patient with acute vertigo, nystagmus is usually visible with the patient looking straight ahead. If the lesion is peripheral, the fast phase is always away from the affected side. Observed down-beating nystagmus indicates a more serious cause than dizziness. There are a variety of examination maneuvers that can be done in the office to evaluate nystagmus. The Barany or Dix-Hallpike maneuver involves moving the patient rapidly from the sitting to the laying down position with the head tilted downward off the table at 45° and rotated 45° to one side. The test is done for each side. This test is a key diagnostic test for BPPV.[11] A positive Dix-Hallpike test shows a burst of rotational nystagmus, directed toward the dependent ear, indicating BPPV.[1,7] The supine roll test for lateral semicircular canal–related vertigo may be performed in patients with a compatible history but a negative Dix-Hallpike maneuver.[2,11] Hearing loss, suggestive of a peripheral cause of vertigo, can be evaluated by having the patient repeat whispered words and numbers or rubbing fingers together softly. The Weber and Rinne tests, done with a tuning fork, are used to distinguish conductive and sensorineural hearing loss.[11] The head impulse test is done to investigate the integrity of the peripheral vestibular system. It is performed by instructing the patient to keep his or her eyes on a distant target. The head is turned quickly by the examiner about 15° with the starting position about 10° from straight ahead. The normal response is that the eyes remain on target. The abnormal response is that the eyes are dragged off target by the head turn (in one direction) followed by a saccade back to the target after the head turn. If the test is normal in patients with sustained vertigo, the peripheral system is normal and central disease should be expected. This test is useful for patients with prolonged vertigo. If the episodes are brief, then BPPV is more likely and the Dix-Hallpike maneuver is more useful.[11,48] Caloric testing is the gold standard but can be extremely uncomfortable and is usually reserved for the vestibular laboratory. The mnemonic COWS is used to describe the direction of the fast component of nystagmus: cold–opposite warm–same.

### Presyncope/Syncope

Presyncope usually occurs when the patient is standing or seated upright and not supine. If presyncope occurs when the patient is supine, then a cardiac arrhythmia should be suspected. Orthostatic hypotension, cardiac arrhythmias, and vasovagal attacks are some of the more common causes of presyncope. An electrocardiogram can correlate symptoms with a dysrhythmia.[11] Orthostatic vital signs are useful in determining this very common cause of dizziness. A systolic blood pressure decrease of 20 mm Hg, a diastolic blood pressure decrease of 10 mm Hg, or a pulse increase of 30 beats per minute on standing indicates orthostatic hypotension. It is important to note the patient's hydration status because signs and symptoms of dizziness can simply be an early sign of dehydration.[7,49,50]

### Disequilibrium

Patients with signs and symptoms of disequilibrium require a thorough and focused neurologic examination with careful observation of gait.[11]

The patient should make several right angle turns while walking without assistance. If dizziness appears during this maneuver, the patient with multiple sensory deficits experiences immediate relief by touching another person's hand or the wall (a maneuver providing additional sensory information that helps resolve the unsteadiness).[5] Further tests for disequilibrium include a Romberg test, standing balanced with eyes open and closed, and an examination for sensory loss in the legs. These tests are for proprioceptive loss and would indicate a peripheral neuropathy. An eye examination with visual acuity testing can assess for causes of visual loss (eg, cataracts).[5]

### Nonspecific

There are no physical signs that are diagnostic of nonspecific dizziness. Purposeful hyperventilation is one method to confirm that diagnosis. The patient is coached to hyperventilate until dizzy to see if the dizziness mimics prior spontaneously occurring symptoms. If nystagmus is seen, the diagnosis is a vestibular lesion, not hyperventilation.[11]

## DIAGNOSIS

Differentiating the diagnosis begins with clarifying the category of dizziness. Initially, it should be determined if the patient is experiencing peripheral or central vertigo. Peripheral vertigo presents with an increased presence of nausea, a negative neurologic examination, and position-related changes. Classic symptoms of central vestibular disorders include associated neurologic findings and/or vertigo that is not position related. Disequilibrium is often obvious based on history; however, if the history is unclear, the evaluation shifts to multifactorial impairment, particularly visual and peripheral sensory function. The most common symptom that indicates cardiovascular involvement is lightheadedness, pointing to cardiac dysrhythmias, orthostatic hypotension, and vasovagal response. Nonspecific dizziness is most often due to psychological causes (eg, anxiety and hyperventilation).[7,10,13,14]

## DIAGNOSTIC TESTING

Diagnostic tests should be ordered for patients who have abnormal findings on physical examination that may indicate a serious cause of dizziness.[1,11] Routine laboratory testing should be completed to evaluate for suspected comorbid conditions.[7,51] Findings suggestive of a central cause of dizziness should prompt consideration of MRI or computed tomographic (CT) scanning. In acute sustained vertigo, MRI or CT scanning should be performed urgently to rule out a vascular event in patients who have headache, vascular risk factors, or an examination that is not completely typical of a peripheral vestibulopathy. It is especially important for patients who have prominent stroke risk factors to obtain a CT scan or MRI.[11,47,52,53] For all patients complaining of dizziness, the low prevalence of serious disorders should be balanced against the need for specialized testing. For brain imaging, the procedures of choice are MRI and magnetic resonance angiography. Audiometry is more sensitive than office testing to detect hearing loss but the audiometric battery is not truly diagnostic of a specific disorder independently of other factors.[54,55] Other specialized testing can include electronystagmography and videonystagmography.[54,56]

## SUMMARY

Patients presenting to primary care with complaints of dizziness are common. Differentiating the cause of dizziness can be made easier by considering 4 main categories of dizziness: vertigo, presyncope/syncope, disequilibrium, and nonspecific symptoms. Differentials should immediately include the most common causes of dizziness, such as BPPV and orthostatic hypotension. Diagnostic tests should be ordered for patients who have abnormal findings on physical examination that may indicate a more serious cause of dizziness. Nystagmus represents the physical manifestation of a patient's complaint of vertigo. Other neurologic symptoms, numbness, weakness, pronounced gait impairment, diplopia, and dysarthria point to a central cause of vertigo. Presyncope/syncope is primarily cardiovascular in origin and requires specific testing for orthostatic hypotension and cardiac dysrhythmias. Disequilibrium involves multisensory defects and requires evaluation and testing of multiple systems to form a cumulative list of deficits. Nonspecific dizziness rarely shows signs that are diagnostic other than purposeful testing for hyperventilation. Nonspecific dizziness has been shown to be primarily psychogenic in origin.

## REFERENCES

1. Howell Collie MJ, Ramsey AR. Differentiating benign paroxysmal vertigo from other causes of dizziness. J Nurse Pract 2014;10(6):393–400.
2. Bhattacharyya N, Baugh RF, Orvidas L, et al. Clinical practice guideline: benign paroxysmal positional vertigo. Otolaryngol Head Neck Surg 2008;139:S47–81.
3. Zhao JG, Piccirillo JF, Spitznagal EL, et al. Predictive capability of historical data for diagnosis of dizziness. Otol Neurotol 2011;32(2):284–90.
4. Neuhauser HK, Lempert T. Vertigo: epidemiologic aspects. Semin Neurol 2009; 29(5):473–81.
5. Molnar A, McGee S. Diagnosing and treating dizziness. Med Clin North Am 2014; 39(3):583–96.
6. Herr RD, Zun L, Mathews JJ. A directed approach to the dizzy patient. Ann Emerg Med 1989;18:664–72.
7. Saccomano SJ. Dizziness, vertigo and presyncope: what's the difference? Nurse Pract 2012;37(12):46–52.
8. Navi BB, Kamel H, Shah MP, et al. Rate and predictors of the serious neurologic causes of dizziness in the emergency department. Mayo Clin Proc 2012;87:1080–8.
9. Kerber KA, Burke JF, Skolarus LE, et al. Use of BPPV processes in emergency department dizziness presentations: a population-based study. Otolaryngol Head Neck Surg 2013;148:425–30.
10. Labuguen RH. Initial evaluation of vertigo. Am Fam Physician 2006;73(2):244–51.
11. Branch WT, Barton JS. Approach to the patient with dizziness. UpToDate. Philadelphia: Wolters Kluwer Health; 2014. topic 5099(version 11.0):1–8.
12. Katsarkas A. Dizziness in the aging: the clinical experience. Geriatrics 2008; 63(11):18–20.
13. Delaney KA. Bedside diagnosis of vertigo: value of the history and neurologic examination. Acad Emerg Med 2003;10(12):1388–95.
14. Kline C. Vertigo, part 1: PNS, CNS causes and red flags. J Amer Chiropr Assoc 2008;45(7):2–7.
15. Nadeau S. Dizziness, vertigo, presyncope, syncope and disequilibrium. The University of Florida website. Available at: http://medinfo.ufl.edu: 8050/year3/ neurology/Dizziness.pdf. Accessed September 12, 2014.
16. Marques PS, Perez-Fernandez N. Bedside vestibular examination in patients with unilateral definite Meniere's disease. Acta Otolaryngol 2012;132:498–504.
17. Rauch SD, Merchant SN, Thedinger BA, et al. Meniere's syndrome and endolymphatic hydrops. Double-blind temporal bone study. Ann Otol Rhinol Laryngol 1989;98:873–83.
18. Nelson JA, Viirre E. The clinical differentiation of cerebellar infarction from common vertigo syndromes. West J Emerg Med 2009;10:273–7.
19. Strupp M, Brandt T. Peripheral vestibular disorders. Curr Opin Neurol 2013;26: 81–9.
20. Desmond AL. Dizziness reference guide. Chatham (IL): Micromedical Technologies; 2009.
21. Grimby A, Rosenthal V. Health related quality of life and dizziness in old age. Gerontology 1995;41:286.
22. Hillen ME, Wagner ML, Sage JI. "Subclinical" orthostatic hypotension is associated with dizziness in elderly patients with Parkinson's disease. Arch Phys Med Rehabil 1996;77:710.
23. Drachman DA, Hart CW. An approach to the dizzy patient. Neurology 1972;22: 323–34.

24. Nedzelski JM, Barber HO, McIlmoyl L. Diagnosis in a dizzy unit. J Otolaryngol 1986;15:101.
25. Rosenthal V, Johansson G, Orndahl G. Otoneurologic and audiologic findings in fibromyalgia. Scand J Rehabil Med 1996;28:225.
26. Lanska DJ. Clinical summary: dizziness. Neurology Medlink. Available at: http://www.Medlink.com/medlinkcontent.asp. Accessed September 12, 2014.
27. Garcia FV. Disequilibrium and it's management in elderly patients. Int Tinnitus J 2009;15(1):83–90.
28. Sloane P, Blazer D, George LK, et al. Dizziness in a community elderly population. J Am Geriatr Soc 1989;37:101–8.
29. Jaap AJ, Jones GC, McCrimmon RJ, et al. Perceived symptoms of hypoglycemia in elderly type 2 diabetic patients treated with insulin. Diabet Med 1998; 15:398.
30. McKiernan JM, Lowe FC. Side effects of terazosin in the treatment of symptomatic benign prostatic hyperplasia. South Med J 1997;90:509.
31. Coupland NJ, Bell CJ, Potokar JP. Serotonin reuptake inhibitor withdrawal. J Clin Psychopharmacol 1996;16:356.
32. Bedard J. Dizziness and syncope. Available at: http://www.lemieuxbedard.com/emc/files/Dizziness_Syncope.pdf. Accessed September 12, 2014.
33. Staab JP, Ruckenstein MJ. Expanding the differential diagnosis of chronic dizziness. Arch Otolaryngol Head Neck Surg 2007;133(2):170–6.
34. Kroenke K, Lucas CA, Rosenberg ML, et al. Causes of persistent dizziness. A prospective study of 100 patients in ambulatory care. Ann Intern Med 1992; 117:898.
35. Ponka D, Kirlew M. Top 10 differential diagnosis in family medicine: vertigo and dizziness. Canadian Family Physician. Available at: http://www.familymedicine.Uottawa.ca/assets/documents/undergrad/top10_Differential_Diagnosis_In_Primary_Care.pdf. Accessed September 14, 2014.
36. Chan Y. Differential diagnosis of dizziness. Curr Opin Otolaryngol Head Neck Surg 2009;17:200–3.
37. Cherchi M, Hain TC. Migraine-associated vertigo. Otolaryngol Clin North Am 2011;44(2):367–75.
38. Sloane PD, Dallara J, Roach C, et al. Management of dizziness in primary care. J Am Board Fam Pract 1994;7:1.
39. Alvord LS, Herr RD. ENG in the emergency room: subtest results in acutely dizzy patients. J Am Acad Audiol 1994;5:384.
40. Madlon-Kay DJ. Evaluation and outcome of the dizzy patient. J Fam Pract 1985; 21:109.
41. Moya A, Sutton R, Ammiriti F, et al. for European Society of Cardiology. Guidelines for the diagnosis and management of syncope (version 2009). Available at: http://www.escardio.org/guidelines-surveys/esc-guidelines/pages/syncope.aspx. Accessed September 14, 2014.
42. Venugopal D, Jhanjee R, Benditt DG. Current management of syncope: focus on drug therapy. Am J Cardiovasc Drugs 2007;7(6):399–411.
43. Thijs RD, Bloem BR, van Dijk JG. Falls, faints, fits and funny turns. J Neurol 2009; 256(2):155–67.
44. Samuels MA, Pomerantz BJ, Sadow PM. Case records of the Massachusetts General Hospital. Case 14-2010. A 54-year-old woman with dizziness and falls. N Engl J Med 2010;362(19):1815–23.
45. Jahn K, Zwergal A, Schniepp R. Gait disturbance in old age. Dtsch Arztebl Int 2010;107(17):306–15.

46. Thanavaro JL. Evaluation and management of syncope. Clinical Scholars Review 2009;2(2):67–77.
47. Stanton VA, Hsieh YH, Camargo CA Jr, et al. Overreliance on symptom quality in diagnosing dizziness: results of a multicenter survey of emergency physicians. Mayo Clin Proc 2007;82:1319.
48. Sloane PD. Evaluation and management of dizziness in the older patient. Clin Geriatr Med 1996;12:785.
49. Kerber KA. Vertigo and dizziness in the emergency department. Emerg Med Clin North Am 2009;27(1):39–50.
50. Becker JA, Stewart LK. Heat-related illness. Am Fam Physician 2011;83(11): 1325–30.
51. Dinces E, Rauch S. Meniere's disease. Philadelphia: Wolters Kluwer Health. Available at: http://www.UpToDate.com/contents/menieres-disease. Accessed September 15, 2014.
52. Skiendzielewski JJ, Martyak G. The weak and dizzy patient. Ann Emerg Med 1980;9:353.
53. Yardley L, Owen N, Nazareth I, et al. Panic disorder with agoraphobia associated with dizziness: characteristic symptoms and psychosocial sequelae. J Nerv Ment Dis 2001;189:321.
54. Furman JM, Barton JS. Approach to the patient with vertigo. UpTo Date. Philadelphia: Wolters Kluwer Health; 2014. Topic Key= Neur: 1–20. Available at: http://www.UpToDate.com/contents/approach-to-the-patient-with-vertigo.
55. Johnson EW. Auditory findings in 200 cases of acoustic neuromas. Arch Otolaryngol 1968;88:598.
56. Hoffman RM, Einstadter D, Kroenke K. Evaluating dizziness. Am J Med 1999;107: 468.

# Medication- and Toxin-Induced Neurologic Syndromes

Cheryl Basden, DO, MBA

## KEYWORDS

• Tremor • Confusion • Seizure • Toxicity • Chemical exposure

## KEY POINTS

• Frequently, patients present to practitioners with various neurologic signs and symptoms that do not fit into a neat diagnostic package.
• The possibility of medication- or toxin-induced neurologic causes must be considered.
• Although only approximately 2% to 4% of patients have medication or toxin-induced neurologic syndrome, including it in the differential diagnosis may help resolve symptoms.

Medication- and toxin-induced neurologic syndrome is a combination of several symptoms that are induced either by the exposure to or withdrawal of various medications or by toxins. Patients present with a variety of neurologic signs and symptoms (**Table 1**), which are sometimes difficult to fit into a nice, neat diagnostic package. Although only approximately 2% to 4% of the patients have neuropathies associated with medications or toxins, this possibility should definitely be considered as part of the differential diagnosis because the symptoms may be reversible.[1] Therefore, it is imperative to understand how to formulate a comprehensive treatment approach for these patients.

The term *neuropathy* refers to a condition of the nervous system: "Toxic neuropathy refers to neuropathy caused by drug ingestion, drug or chemical abuse, or industrial chemical exposure from the workplace or the environment."[2,3] The ingested drugs can be those obtained by prescription or those ingested socially, including chemicals such as alcohol (**Table 2**).

## SIGNS AND SYMPTOMS

The signs and symptoms of medication- and toxin-induced neurologic syndrome are sometimes different depending on the causative agents and the areas affected. For

Clinical Education, 625 Old Peachtree Road, Suwanee, GA 30025, USA
*E-mail address:* Basdenc@aol.com

Prim Care Clin Office Pract 42 (2015) 259–265
http://dx.doi.org/10.1016/j.pop.2015.01.002     **primarycare.theclinics.com**
0095-4543/15/$ – see front matter © 2015 Elsevier Inc. All rights reserved.

| Table 1 | |
|---|---|
| Medication- and toxin-induced signs and symptoms | |
| Characteristics | Symptoms |
| Tremors | Involuntary shaking movement in parts of or the entire body |
| Seizures | Mental status changes, memory loss, and/or visual problems |
| | Jerking movements or momentary loss of awareness |
| Tinnitus | Noise or ringing in the ears |
| | Bilateral or unilateral, continuous or intermittent |
| Polyneuropathy | Sensory changes, numbness, weakness, burning, pain |
| | Often starts in the hands and feet and progress upward |
| | Usually bilateral |
| | Can cause reflex impairment |

example, tremors, seizures, tinnitus, and polyneuropathy are some of the associated symptoms that may help identify an insulting agent.

## Types of Tremors

A tremor is an involuntary shaking or movement of a body part or the entire body, and may occur in conjunction with another disease process or alone. The types of tremors are as follows:

- Action (intentional) tremor: noted during intentional movements of the patient
- Postural tremor: noted during attempts to maintain the patient's posture
- Resting tremor (static): noted while the patient is at rest
- Task-specific tremor: noted while the patient is attempting a specific task
- Physiologic tremors: noted in normal individuals commonly in the hands

Physiologic tremors are the most common type of tremor seen in drug-induced cases. An enhanced form of physiologic tremors can be seen with various medications, such as bronchodilators and antidepressants. These tremors usually resolve when use of the causative agent is terminated.

Postural or action tremors can be noted in drug-induced Parkinson disease. They are usually caused by medications such as neuroleptics, lithium, and also by some ß-adrenergic agonists.[4]

Alcohol can cause tremors such as asterixis (a tremor occurring in the hand during wrist extension that resembles a bird flapping its wings). It can also cause cerebellar tremors. Cerebellar tremors are intentional tremors that can be either unilateral or bilateral.[5]

## Seizures

Seizure is "a sudden disruption of the brain's normal electrical activity accompanied by altered consciousness and/or other neurologic and behavioral manifestations."

Causes can be associated with environmental exposure, such as lead poisoning and exposure to organophosphates (eg, pesticides and fertilizers).

Causes can also be from prescription-ingested products, such as tricyclic antidepressants, theophylline, propranolol, and lidocaine, and non–prescription-ingested products, such as caffeine, ethanol, and cocaine.[6]

## Tinnitus

Tinnitus is a disorder described as a ringing in the ear in the absence of actual sound.

This symptom occurs as a side effect of certain medications, known as *ototoxic tinnitus*, or can be associated with sensorineural disorders.

There are 2 types of tinnitus: subjective and objective.

### Subjective
Subjective tinnitus can be caused by ototoxic drugs, such as aspirin and antiarrhythmic medications, or benzodiazepine withdrawal.

### Objective
Objective tinnitus is usually associated with muscle spasms or pulsations.[7,8]

### Polyneuropathy

In acute cases of polyneuropathy, toxin- and drug-induced causes must be entertained. Certain drugs can affect the motor and/or sensory nerves, causing various symptoms, such as

- Motor polyneuropathy: chloroquine
- Distal sensory neuropathy: metronidazole
- Sensorimotor neuropathy: isoniazid

In more chronic cases of polyneuropathy, an alcoholic origin must be included in the differential diagnosis.[9]

Elevated blood concentration, associated comorbidities, and genetic predisposition may make any medication, including antibiotics, potentially neurotoxic.

Cephalosporins, although commonly used antibiotics, have been known to cause neurotoxicity. This association has been more apparent in patients with comorbidities, such as renal disease. "The typical time period for encephalopathy induced by cephalosporin use is a latency of 1 to 10 days following start of medication, and resolution in 2 to 7 days following discontinuation."[10]

## PHYSICAL EXAMINATION

Complaints by the patient may include visual disturbances, tachycardia, orthostatic changes, excessive sweating, diarrhea, tinnitus, and tremors.

It is important to identify whether the symptoms are acute or chronic. The onset of symptoms may coincide with medication changes or recent environmental exposure.

Vital signs should be observed carefully because the risk of medication-induced toxicity increases with age, and alterations in blood pressure can indicate cardiac diseases or comorbidities, which can cause individuals to be more prone to medication toxicity.

## NEUROLOGIC EXAMINATION

Both sensory and motor dysfunction might be noted:

- An abnormal gait may signify motor dysfunction.
- Sensory dysfunction may appear in a "stocking-glove" pattern.

The nerve cell is divided into the axon, myelin sheath, and cell body, any of which can be affected. Toxin-induced damage usually causes a distal axonopathy or dying-back neuropathy.[2]

During the neurologic examination, noting the specific findings may help pinpoint the affected area when evaluating for polyneuropathy.

**Table 2**
Clinical syndromes and potential chemical etiologic agents

| Category | Clinical Syndrome | Potential Chemical Etiologic Agent |
|---|---|---|
| Cholinergic crisis | • Salivation, diarrhea, lacrimation, bronchorrhea, diaphoresis, and/or urination<br>• Miosis, fasciculations, weakness, bradycardia or tachycardia, hypotension or hypertension, altered mental status, and/or seizures | • Nicotine[a]<br>• Organophosphate insecticides[a]<br>  ◦ Decreased acetylcholinesterase-teras activity<br>• Carbamate insecticides<br>• Cholinergic syndrome (eg, physostigmine) |
| Generalized muscle rigidity | • Seizure-like generalized muscle contractions or painful spasms (neck and limbs) and usually tachycardia and hypertension | • Strychnine<br>  ◦ Intact sensorium |
| Oropharyngeal pain and ulcerations | • Lip, mouth, and pharyngeal ulcerations and burning pain | • Paraquat[a]<br>  ◦ Dyspnea and hemoptysis secondary to pulmonary edema or hemorrhage; can progress to pulmonary fibrosis over days to weeks<br>• Diquat<br>• Caustics (ie, acids and alkalis)<br>• Inorganic mercuric salts<br>• Mustards (eg, sulfur) |
| Cellular hypoxia | • Mild: nausea, vomiting, and headache<br>• Severe: altered mental status, dyspnea, hypotension, seizures, and metabolic acidosis | • Cyanide (eg, hydrogen cyanide gas or sodium cyanide)<br>  ◦ Bitter almond odor[b]<br>• Sodium monofluoroacetate[a]<br>  ◦ Hypocalcemia or hypokalemia<br>• Carbon monoxide<br>• Hydrogen sulfide<br>• Sodium azide<br>• Methemoglobinemia (cetacaine, benzocaine, dapsone, nitrite) |

| | | |
|---|---|---|
| Peripheral neuropathy and/or neurocognitive effects | • Peripheral neuropathy signs and symptoms: muscle weakness and atrophy, "glove and stocking" sensory loss, and depressed or absent deep tendon reflexes<br>• Neurocognitive effects: memory loss, delirium, ataxia, and/or encephalopathy | • Mercury (organic)<br>  ○ Visual disturbances, paresthesias, and/or ataxia<br>• Arsenic (inorganic)[a]<br>  ○ Delirium and/or peripheral neuropathy<br>• Thallium<br>  ○ Delirium and/or peripheral neuropathy<br>• Lead<br>  ○ Encephalopathy<br>• Acrylamide<br>  ○ Encephalopathy and/or peripheral neuropathy |
| Severe gastrointestinal illness, dehydration | • Abdominal pain, vomiting, profuse diarrhea (possibly bloody), and hypotension, possibly followed by multi-system organ failure | • Arsenic[a]<br>• Ricin[a]<br>  ○ Inhalation is an additional route of exposure; severe respiratory illness possible<br>• Colchicine<br>• Barium<br>  ○ Hypokalemia common |

Not intended as a complete differential diagnosis for each syndrome or a list of all chemicals that might be used in a covert chemical release.

[a] Potential agents for a covert chemical release based on historic use (ie, intentional or inadvertent use, high toxicity, and/or ease of availability).

[b] Unreliable sign.

From Centers for Disease Control and Prevention. Recognition of illness associated with exposure to chemical agents—United States, 2003. MMWR Morb Mortal Wkly Rep 2003;52(39):938–40. Available at: http://www.cdc.gov/mmwr/preview/mmwrhtml/mm5239a3.htm.

After performing a thorough history and physical examination, medication- and toxin-induced effects should be differentiated from other complicating chronic diseases.

Following are some other diagnoses that could be considered:

- Diabetic neuropathy
- Liver disease
- Vitamin deficiency
- Infection
- Cancer
- Toxins (medication-related or environmental)
- Stoke
- Sarcoidosis
- Lyme disease

A host of others differential diagnoses can be included, depending on the history and physical examination.

As with most medical conditions, the physician must narrow down the differential diagnosis. The first approach usually includes laboratory tests, which are the least invasive, but still useful.

### Laboratory Results

Laboratory assessment should include a complete blood cell count, hepatitis C and HIV serologies, and sometimes cerebrospinal fluid analysis to evaluate for infectious causes.

A comprehensive metabolic panel, vitamin B levels, and urine with microalbumin can help establish the differential diagnosis, which may include diabetes, renal failure, endocrine diseases, and cancer.

Ancillary laboratory tests could include the cryoglobins test (which evaluates disorders associated with abnormal protein levels) and electrophoresis.[11]

Other laboratory tests can be performed to help either confirm or eliminate various diagnoses, depending on the high level of suspicion.

### Additional Testing

Additional tests may include electrodiagnostic testing along with imaging.

- "Electrodiagnostic testing can document the presence of peripheral nerve disease, define the distribution and pattern of various sensory and motor fibers and characterize the underlying pathologic processes."[12]
- Electroencephalography in patients suspected of having toxic metabolic encephalopathy may show slowing and triphasic waves.[10]
- Electromyography can help evaluate neuropathy.
- MRI and computed tomography scans can show changes in the cerebral hemisphere and white matter, which can help in diagnosing the process of myelinopathy.[13]

### SUMMARY

Patients frequently present to practitioners with various neurologic signs and symptoms that do not fit into a nice, neat diagnostic package. The possibility of medication- or toxin-induced neurologic causes must be considered. Although only approximately 2% to 4% of patients have medication or toxin-induced neurologic syndrome, including it in the differential diagnosis may help resolve symptoms.

## REFERENCES

1. Weimer LH. Drug-induced neuropathies. Available at: http://www.medlink.com/medlinkcontent.asp. Accessed February 2, 2013.
2. Rutchik JS, Ramachandran T, Centers for Disease Control and Prevention (CDC). Toxic neuropathy. Medscape Medical News 2014.
3. Centers for Disease Control and Prevention. Recognition of illness associated with exposure to chemical agents—United States, 2003. MMWR Morb Mortal Wkly Rep 2003;52(39):938–40. Available at: http://www.cdc.gov/mmwr/preview/mmwrhtml/mm5239a3.htm.
4. Ahmed A, Sweeney P. Tremors. Available at: http://www.clevelandclinicmeded.com/medicalpubs/diseasemanagement/nerology/tremors/.
5. Seeberger LC. Cerebellar tremors definition and treatment. The Colorado Neurological Institute Review. 2005.
6. Goetz CG, Meisel E. Biological neurotoxins. Neurol Clin 2000;18(3):719–40.
7. "Tinnitus" American Academy of Otolaryngology- Head and Neck Surgery 2012-04-03. Available at: http://www.entnet.org/HealthInformation/tinnitus.cfm. Accessed October 26, 2012.
8. Brown RD, Penny JE, Henley CM, et al. Ototoxic drugs and noise. Ciba Found Symp 1981;85:151–71.
9. Routledge PA, Lane RJ. Drug-induced neurological disorders. BMJ 1979;863.
10. Grill MF, Maganti RK. Neurotoxic effects associated with antibiotic use: management considerations. Br J Clin Pharmacol 2011;72(3):381–93.
11. England JD, Gronseth GS, Franklin G, et al. Distal symmetrical polyneuropathy: A definition for clinical research. Report of the American Academy of Neurology, the American Association of Electrodiagnostic Medicine, and the American Academy of Physical Medicine and Rehabilitation. Neurology 2005;64(2):199–207.
12. Shields RW Jr, Harris JW, Clark M, et al. Mononeuropathy in sickle cell anemia: anatomical and pathophysiological basis for its rarity. Muscle Nerve 1991;14(4):370–4.
13. Schprecher D, Mehta L. The syndrome of delayed post-hypoxic leukoencephalopathy. NeuroRehabilitation 2010;26:65–72. Available at: http://www.ncbi.nlm.nih.gov/pmc/articles/PMC2835522/.

Printed and bound by CPI Group (UK) Ltd, Croydon, CR0 4YY

03/10/2024

01040489-0011